Neurologic Emergencies

Guest Editors

ROBERT SILBERGLEIT, MD
ROMERGRYKO G. GEOCADIN, MD

EMERGENCY MEDICINE CLINICS OF NORTH AMERICA

www.emed.theclinics.com

Consulting Editor
AMAL MATTU, MD

February 2009 • Volume 27 • Number 1

SAUNDERS an imprint of ELSEVIER, Inc.

W.B. SAUNDERS COMPANY

A Division of Elsevier Inc.

1600 John F. Kennedy Boulevard ● Suite 1800 ● Philadelphia, Pennsylvania 19103-2899

http://www.theclinics.com

EMERGENCY MEDICINE CLINICS OF NORTH AMERICA Volume 27, Number 1
February 2009 ISSN 0733-8627, ISBN-13: 978-1-4160-6290-5, ISBN-10: 1-4160-6290-4

Editor: Patrick Manley
Developmental Editor: Donald Mumford

Emergency Medicine Clinics of North America (ISSN 0733-8627) is published quarterly by Elsevier Inc., 360 Park Avenue South, New York, NY, 10010-1710. Months of issue are February, May, August, and November. Business and Editorial Offices: 1600 John F. Kennedy Boulevard, Suite 1800, Philadelphia, PA 19103-2899. Customer Service Office: 6277 Sea Harbor Drive, Orlando, FL 32887-4800. Periodicals postage paid at New York, NY, and additional mailing offices. Subscription prices are $118.00 per year (US students), $229.00 per year (US individuals), $373.00 per year (US institutions), $167.00 per year (international students), $328.00 per year (international individuals), $450.00 per year (international institutions), $167.00 per year (Canadian students), $282.00 per year (Canadian individuals), and $450.00 per year (Canadian institutions). International air speed delivery is included in all *Clinics'* subscription prices. All prices are subject to change without notice. **POSTMASTER:** Send address changes to *Emergency Medicine Clinics of North America*, Elsevier Periodicals Customer Service, 11830 Westline Industrial Drive, St. Louis, MO 63146. Customer Service (orders, claims, online, change of address): Elsevier Periodicals Customer Service, 11830 Westline Industrial Drive, St. Louis, MO 63146. Tel: 1-800-654-2452 (U.S. and Canada); 314-453-7041 (outside U.S. and Canada). Fax: 314-453-5170. E-mail: journalscustomerservice-usa@elsevier.com (for print support); journalsonline support-usa@elsevier.com (for online support).

Reprints. For copies of 100 or more of articles in this publication, please contact the Commercial Reprints Department, Elsevier Inc., 360 Park Avenue South, New York, NY 10010-1710. Tel.: 212-633-3812; Fax: 212-462-1935; E-mail: reprints@elsevier.com.

Emergency Medicine Clinics of North America is covered in *MEDLINE/PubMed (Index Medicus), Current Contents/Clinical Medicine, EMBASE/Excerpta Medica, BIOSIS, SciSearch, CINAHL, ISI/BIOMED,* and *Research Alert.*

Printed and bound by CPI Group (UK) Ltd, Croydon, CR0 4YY

Transferred to Digital Print 2011

Contributors

CONSULTING EDITOR

AMAL MATTU, MD, FAAEM, FACEP
Associate Professor and Program Director, Emergency Medicine Residency, University of Maryland School of Medicine, Baltimore, Maryland

GUEST EDITORS

ROBERT SILBERGLEIT, MD
Associated Professor of Emergency Medicine, University of Michigan Neuro Emergencies Research, Ann Arbor, Michigan

ROMERGRYKO G. GEOCADIN, MD
Director, Neurosciences Critical Care Unit, Johns Hopkins Bayview Medical Center; Associate Professor of Neurology, Anesthesiology—Critical Care Medicine and Neurological Surgery, Johns Hopkins University School of Medicine, Baltimore, Maryland

AUTHORS

BENJAMIN S. ABELLA, MD, MPhil
Assistant Professor, Department of Emergency Medicine and Center for Resuscitation Science, University of Pennsylvania, Philadelphia, Pennsylvania

C. JESSICA DINE, MD
Instructor, Department of Medicine, Division of Pulmonary, Allergy and Critical Care, University of Pennsylvania, Philadelphia, Pennsylvania

BENJAMIN WOLKIN FRIEDMAN, MD, MS
Assistant Professor of Emergency Medicine, Department of Emergency Medicine, Albert Einstein College of Medicine, Montefiore Medical Center, Bronx, New York

NINA T. GENTILE, MD
Associate Professor, Department of Emergency Medicine, Temple University School of Medicine; Director, Clinical Research Administration, Health Sciences Center, Temple University, Philadelphia, Pennsylvania

JOSHUA N. GOLDSTEIN, MD, PhD
Instructor of Surgery (Emergency Medicine) at Harvard Medical School, Department of Emergency Medicine, Massachusetts General Hospital, Boston, Massachusetts

DAVID M. GREER, MD, MA
Assistant Professor of Neurology at Harvard Medical School, Department of Neurology, Massachusetts General Hospital, Boston, Massachusetts

BRIAN MITCHELL GROSBERG, MD
Assistant Professor of Neurology, Department of Neurology, Albert Einstein College
of Medicine, Bronx, New York

J. CLAUDE HEMPHILL III, MD, MAS
Associate Professor of Clinical Neurology and Neurological Surgery, University of
California; Director, Neurocritical Care, San Francisco General Hospital, San Francisco,
California

KEVIN A. KERBER, MD
Assistant Professor, Department of Neurology, University of Michigan Health System,
Ann Arbor, Michigan

MARK J. LOWELL, MD
Associate Professor; Medical Director, Survival Flight Department of Emergency
Medicine, University of Michigan, Ann Arbor, Michigan

WILLIAM MEURER, MD
Department of Emergency Medicine, University of Michigan; Department of Neurology,
University of Michigan, Ann Arbor, Michigan

DAN MILLIKAN, MD
Department of Emergency Medicine, University of Michigan, Ann Arbor, Michigan

FADI NAHAB, MD
Instructor, Department of Neurology, Emory University, Atlanta, Georgia

BRIAN RICE, MD
Clinical Lecturer, Department of Emergency Medicine, Hurley Medical Center Division,
University of Michigan, Ann Arbor, Michigan

MICHAEL ROSS, MD
Associate Professor, Department of Emergency Medicine, Emory University, Atlanta,
Georgia

PHILLIP A. SCOTT, MD
Associate Professor, Department of Emergency Medicine, University of Michigan, Ann
Arbor, Michigan

ROBERT SILBERGLEIT, MD
Associated Professor of Emergency Medicine, University of Michigan Neuro Emergencies
Research, Ann Arbor, Michigan

KAREN SIREN, MD
Resident, Emergency Medicine Residency Program, Temple University Hospital,
Philadelphia, Pennsylvania

DAVID SOMAND, MD
Department of Emergency Medicine, University of Michigan, Taubman Center, Ann Arbor,
Michigan

BRADLEY UREN, MD
Clinical Instructor, Department of Emergency Medicine and Survival Flight, University of Michigan, Ann Arbor, Michigan

DOUGLAS B. WHITE, MD, MAS
Assistant Professor of Medicine and Anesthesia, University of California; Director, UCSF Clinical Ethics Core, San Francisco, California

Contents

> In the emergency and critical care setting, a comprehensive and thorough neurologic examination can be impractical. The clinical context should therefore focus the examination on those features relevant to acute diagnosis and management. This article discusses how to direct the history and examination in patients who have focal complaints, possible strokes affecting the anterior or posterior circulations, neck or back pain, neuromuscular complaints, global symptoms, or nonanatomic complaints.

> This article reviews the special questions and issues in critical care transport related specifically to the care of patients who have neurologic emergencies. It first considers potential indications for transport and reviews attempts to create a hierarchical stroke center system akin to that developed for trauma care. It then discusses therapeutic concerns relating to the transport environment and the use of specific interventions, including the effects of end-tidal CO_2 monitoring on intracranial pressure, patient outcomes after traumatic brain injury, and opportunities to initiate therapeutic hypothermia in comatose survivors of cardiac arrest during transport. Finally, the cost of critical care transport of patients who have neurologic emergencies is considered.

> Mortality and morbidity remain high from neurologic emergencies, such as acute stroke, traumatic brain injury, and hypoxic-ischemic encephalopathy after cardiac arrest. Decisions regarding initial aggressiveness of care must be made at the time of presentation, and perceived prognosis is often used as part of this decision-making process. These decisions are predicated on the accuracy of early outcome prediction, however.

Decisions to limit treatment early after neuroemergencies must be balanced with avoidance of self-fulfilling prophecies of poor outcome attributable to clinical nihilism. This article examines the role of prognostication early after neuroemergences, the potential impact of early treatment limitations, and how these may relate to communication with patients and surrogate decision makers in the context of these acute neurologic events.

Understanding three peripheral vestibular disorders—vestibular neuritis, benign paroxysmal positional vertigo, and Meniere's disease—is the key to the evaluation and management of vertigo and dizziness presentations in the emergency department. Each of these benign disorders is a common cause of a broad category of dizziness presentation. In addition, each of these disorders has characteristic features that allow for a bedside diagnosis. An effective strategy for "ruling-out" a serious disorder, such as stroke, is "ruling-in" a peripheral vestibular disorder. In this article a focus is on the key features of these disorders.

Patients who have a transient ischemic attack (TIA) represent a group that may appear well but are at high risk for stroke within 90 days. Management of patients who have a TIA requires an understanding of the short-term risk for stroke to guide acute management and the long-term benefits to medical and surgical therapies. The initial emergency department (ED) evaluation may be supplemented with simple TIA stroke risk scores to estimate short-term stroke risk. The addition of MRI provides yet more information regarding stroke risks, while identifying some specific causes of TIA. Extended testing may not be feasible in the ED, and to address this limitation, new outpatient strategies for patients who have a TIA have been developed, such as the use of an ED observation unit or an outpatient TIA clinic. Although controversy remains in some areas of acute TIA management because of the lack of evidence from controlled trials, evidence from large randomized trials have led to a better understanding of effective measures for the long-term prevention of stroke.

Headache continues to be a frequent cause of emergency department (ED) use, accounting for 2% of all visits. Most of these headaches prove to be benign but painful exacerbations of chronic headache disorders, such as migraine, tension-type, and cluster. The goal of ED management is to provide rapid and quick relief of benign headache, without causing undue side effects, and to recognize headaches with malignant course. Although these headaches have distinct epidemiologies and clinical phenotypes, there is overlapping response to therapy; nonsteroidals, triptans, dihydroergotamine, and the antiemetic dopamine antagonists may play a therapeutic role for each of these acute headaches. This article reviews the diagnostic criteria and management strategies for the primary headache disorders.

Central nervous system infections have long been recognized as among the most devastating of diseases. This article describes the changing pattern and epidemiology of a variety of common central nervous system infections, including meningitis, encephalitis, and brain abscesses, and reviews pathophysiology and the most current approach to clinical diagnosis, treatment, and disposition from the emergency physician perspective.

Current thinking about the acute treatment of status epilepticus (SE) emphasizes a more aggressive clinical approach to this common life-threatening neurologic emergency. In this review, the authors consider four concepts that can accelerate effective treatment of SE. These include (1) updating the definition of SE to make it more clinically relevant, (2) consideration of faster ways to initiate first-line benzodiazepine therapy in the prehospital environment, (3) moving to second-line agents more quickly in refractory status in the emergency department, and (4) increasing detection and treatment of unrecognized nonconvulsive SE in comatose neurologic emergency patients.

Improving the clinical outcomes of stroke patients depends on the adoption of proven new therapies throughout the broader medical community. Approximately 1% of stroke patients in community settings are receiving tissue plasminogen activator (tPA) therapy 12 years after US Food and Drug Administration approval. Knowledge translation, the process by which the results of clinical investigations are adopted by clinicians and incorporated into routine practice, is important but often overlooked. This article reviews the history of tPA use in stroke as a case study of a breakdown of knowledge translation in emergency medicine. It reviews knowledge translation concepts and theory and explores practical community–academic collaborative methods based on these tenets to enhance acute stroke care delivery in the community setting.

This review briefly discusses induced therapeutic hypothermia (TH), which represents the intentional induction of a lowered core body temperature of 35 °C or less. The focus is on resuscitative or postarrest hypothermia, the data that support it, and the practical issues pertaining to TH implementation.

The interaction between glycemic control and critical neurologic illness and injury is complex. Hyperglycemia can be either the cause or the result of severe brain injury. Hyperglycemia in acute neurologic injury is associated with worse neurologic outcomes. Demographic patterns, including an aging population and shifts in racial and ethnic representation, contribute to the increasing prevalence of hyperglycemia and diabetes among victims of the most common neurologic emergencies. This article reviews the epidemiology of the problem, relevant pathophysiology, the use of tight glycemic control therapy in other populations, and the potential for tight glycemic control as a way to improve outcomes after acute neurologic illness and injury.

RELATED INTEREST

Neurologic Clinics, Volume 26, Issue 2, Pages 345–616 (May 2008)
Neurologic Critical Care
R.D. Stevens and R.G. Geocadin, *Guest Editors*
www.neurologic.theclinics.com

THE CLINICS ARE NOW AVAILABLE ONLINE!

Access your subscription at:
www.theclinics.com

GOAL STATEMENT

The goal of *Emergency Medicine Clinics of North America* is to keep practicing physicians up to date with current clinical practice in emergency medicine by providing timely articles reviewing the state of the art in patient care.

ACCREDITATION

The *Emergency Medical Clinics of North America* is planned and implemented in accordance with the Essential Areas and Policies of the Accreditation Council for Continuing Medical Education (ACCME) through the joint sponsorship of the University of Virginia School of Medicine and Elsevier. The University of Virginia School of Medicine is accredited by the ACCME to provide continuing medical education for physicians.

The University of Virginia School of Medicine designates this educational activity for a maximum of 15 *AMA PRA Category 1 Credits*™. Physicians should only claim credit commensurate with the extent of their participation in the activity.

The American Medical Association has determined that physicians not licensed in the US who participate in this CME activity are eligible for *AMA PRA Category 1 Credits*™.

Credit can be earned by reading the text material, taking the CME examination online at http://www.theclinics. com/home/cme, and completing the evaluation. After taking the test, you will be required to review any and all incorrect answers. Following completion of the test and evaluation, your credit will be awarded and you may print your certificate.

FACULTY DISCLOSURE/CONFLICT OF INTEREST

The University of Virginia School of Medicine, as an ACCME accredited provider, endorses and strives to comply with the Accreditation Council for Continuing Medical Education (ACCME) Standards of Commercial Support, Commonwealth of Virginia statutes, University of Virginia policies and procedures, and associated federal and private regulations and guidelines on the need for disclosure and monitoring of proprietary and financial interests that may affect the scientific integrity and balance of content delivered in continuing medical education activities under our auspices.

The University of Virginia School of Medicine requires that all CME activities accredited through this institution be developed independently and be scientifically rigorous, balanced and objective in the presentation/discussion of its content, theories and practices.

All authors/editors participating in an accredited CME activity are expected to disclose to the readers relevant financial relationships with commercial entities occurring within the past 12 months (such as grants or research support, employee, consultant, stock holder, member of speakers bureau, etc.). The University of Virginia School of Medicine will employ appropriate mechanisms to resolve potential conflicts of interest to maintain the standards of fair and balanced education to the reader. Questions about specific strategies can be directed to the Office of Continuing Medical Education, University of Virginia School of Medicine, Charlottesville, Virginia.

The faculty and staff of the University of Virginia Office of Continuing Medical Education have no financial affiliations to disclose.

The authors/editors listed below have identified no professional or financial affiliations for themselves or their spouse/partner:
Constance Jessica Dine, MD; Benjamin Wolkin Friedman, MD, MS; David M. Greer, MD, MA; Kevin A. Kerber, MD; Mark J. Lowell, MD; Patrick Manley (Acquisitions Editor); Amal Mattu, MD, FAAEM, FACEP (Consulting Editor); William J. Meurer, MD; Daniel John Millikan, MD; Fadi Nahab, MD; Brian Rice, MD; Michael A. Ross, MD; Phillip A. Scott, MD; Robert Silbergleit, MD (Guest Editor); Karen Siren, MD; David M. Somand, MD; Bradley Uren, MD; Bill Woods, MD (Test Author); and Douglas B. White, MD, MAS.

The authors/editors listed below have identified the following professional or financial affiliations for themselves of their spouse/partner:
Benjamin S. Abella, MD, MPhil has received grants from National Institutes of Health, Philips Medical Systems, and Cardiac Science Corporation, is a consultant for Philips Healthcare, receives honoraria from Philips Healthcare, Alsius Corporation, Medivance Corporation, and Gaymar Corporation, and received equipment from Laerdal Medical Corporation.
Nina T. Gentile, MD an industry funded research/investigator for Sanofi.
Romergryko G. Geocadin, MD (Guest Editor) serves on the Speakers Bureau for Medicines Company.
Joshua N. Goldstein, MD, PhD is a consultant for CSL Behring and Genentech.
Brian Mitchell Grosberg, MD is an industry funded research/investigator for GSK, Merck, Capnia, Advanced Bionics, Allergan, Minster Pharmaceuticals, and Endo, and serves on the Speakers Bureau for GSK and Merck.
J. Claude Hemphill III, MD, MAS is a consultant for Novo Nordisk and UCB Pharma, serves on the Advisory Board for Innercool and Ornim, and has received research support from Novo Nordisk.

Disclosure of Discussion of Non-FDA Approved Uses for Pharmaceutical Products and/or Medical Devices
The University of Virginia School of Medicine, as an ACCME provider, requires that all faculty presenters identify and disclose any off-label uses for pharmaceutical and medical device products. The University of Virginia School of Medicine recommends that each physician fully review all the available data on new products or procedures prior to clinical use.

TO ENROLL

To enroll in the *Emergency Medicine Clinics of North America* Continuing Medical Education program, call customer service at 1-800-654-2452 or visit us online at www.theclinics.com/home/cme. The CME program is available to subscribers for an additional fee of $195.00.

Foreword

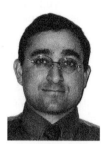

Amal Mattu, MD, FAAEM, FACEP
Consulting Editor

For generations of physicians, the brain has long been considered the "black box" of the human body. Physicians' inability to understand the inner workings of the brain has limited our ability to treat many common neurologic conditions. As a result, for many years there were significant portions of neurology that were simply focused on supportive therapy and rehabilitation: in essence, "damage control." However, recent advances in neuroimaging, increased understanding of neuropathology, and advances in neuropharmacology have dramatically changed the field of neurology from one in which a diagnosis was used to determine the type of supportive therapy, to one in which the diagnosis is used to determine immediate life- or limb-saving therapy. Localization of the lesion is no longer a leisurely academic activity that takes place in the "team room" the day after admission; it instead is a time-sensitive skill that often determines emergent therapy. Emergency neurology is becoming a subspecialty, certainly an academic niche, in and of itself for emergency physicians, neurologists, radiologists, and intensivists—and deservedly so. Many hospitals now recognize that most emergent neurologic conditions are optimally managed by a dedicated multidisciplinary team.

In this issue of *Emergency Medicine Clinics of North America*, Guest Editors Drs. Silbergleit and Geocadin have assembled a multidisciplinary team to educate us about the latest advances and approaches to neurologic emergencies. Perhaps the most important of the articles comes early in the issue and addresses rapid focused neurologic assessment. This certainly is a topic that should be read by all emergency medicine trainees and practitioners. Common and vexing complaints such as vertigo, dizziness, and headache are then addressed. Reasons for misdiagnosis of these complaints are reviewed, and rational approaches to the workup are discussed. The latest pharmacologic treatments for high-risk conditions such as status epilepticus and central nervous system infections are addressed as well. Hot topics in emergency medicine, such as ischemic stroke, transient ischemic attack, glycemic control, and therapeutic hypothermia, are discussed at length. Additionally, the ever-controversial issue of thrombolysis in stroke is reviewd in a balanced and evidence-based manner. The authors also address systems issues, such as critical care transport and community delivery of tPA, for those readers involved in health policy matters and public education.

Emerg Med Clin N Am 27 (2009) xv–xvi
doi:10.1016/j.emc.2008.12.002
0733-8627/08/$ – see front matter © 2009 Elsevier Inc. All rights reserved.

emed.theclinics.com

The guest editors and authors are to be commended for their hard work. This issue represents an invaluable addition to emergency neurology literature. The text is an important step toward helping those of us in emergency medicine open up that "black box" to see its contents more clearly and deliver the most up-to-date therapies to our patients who suffer from acute neurologic conditions.

Amal Mattu, MD, FAAEM, FACEP
Associate Professor and Program Director
Emergency Medicine Residency
University of Maryland School of Medicine
110 S. Paca Street, 6th Floor, Suite 200
Baltimore, MD 21201, USA

E-mail address:
amattu@smail.umaryland.edu (A. Mattu)

Preface

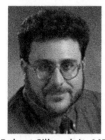 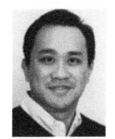

Robert Silbergleit, MD   Romergryko G. Geocadin, MD
Guest Editors

Neurological emergencies are a common presentation, with more than 1 in 14 visits to the emergency department resulting from symptoms referable to the nervous system or in diagnoses of a nonpsychiatric disease of the nervous system or neurotrauma. Moreover, neurological emergencies represent a huge burden of disease. Eight conditions (acute ischemic stroke, intracerebral hemorrhage, subarachnoid hemorrhage, traumatic brain injury, spinal cord injury, bacterial meningitis, status epilepticus, and hypoxic ischemic encephalopathy) affect 1.1 million patients per year and are responsible for 250,000 deaths annually in the United States. Patients with these conditions who live have substantial functional impairment. Collectively, these neurologic conditions are the leading cause of permanent adult disability.

Until recently, emergency and critical care aspects of these neurologic disorders were not a substantial part of the training or practice mindset of any specialty groups. Over the past several years, however, parallel efforts within emergency medicine and neurocritical care have focused on and developed expertise in the emergency care of patients with critical neurological illnesses and injuries. Within emergency medicine, there has been increased attention paid to the neurological emergencies in the specialty's curriculum and residency training, and neurological emergencies have become a major focus of NIH clinical research funding for investigators in emergency medicine. From a broad range of specialties, particularly neurology, anesthesiology, internal medicine, and neurosurgery, evolved a group of specialists focusing on the life-threatening conditions of neurologic disease that has formally been amalgamated into the Neurocritical Care Society (www.neurocriticalcare.org). Perhaps not surprisingly, specialists in emergency medicine and neurocritical care have a lot in common, including the skills and a penchant for rapid patient assessment and early intervention. Working together from these new disciplinary bases, all of us have an opportunity to improve the care of patients with neurological emergencies in ways that were not possible before. This is an exciting time.

In a sense, this issue *of Emergency Medicine Clinics of North America* is a manifestation of the mergence of emergency and critical care neurology. The authors of each article provide expertise from both emergency medicine and acute care neurology and have focused on the approach to patients with neurological conditions, rather than on

Emerg Med Clin N Am 27 (2009) xvii–xviii
doi:10.1016/j.emc.2008.12.003
0733-8627/08/$ – see front matter © 2009 Elsevier Inc. All rights reserved.

static facts about the pathology itself. In so doing, the articles are relevant to both academics and those in community practice, as well as to practitioners of emergency medicine and acute care neurology. To some, these articles may convey new ideas or practices, while others may look to them for a consolidated view of management strategies of which they were already aware, but there is something here for everybody. It is fortunate that patients with neurological emergencies are finally getting the attention they are due, and we feel fortunate to have helped assemble these articles in this emerging field.

Robert Silbergleit, MD
Department of Emergency Medicine
University of Michigan Neuro Emergencies Research
24 Frank Lloyd Wright Drive, Lobby H, Suite 3100
PO Box 381, Ann Arbor, MI 48106

Romergryko G. Geocadin, MD
Neurosciences Critical Care Unit
Johns Hopkins Bayview Medical Center
Baltimore, MD

Johns Hopkins University School of Medicine
600 North Wolfe Street–Mayer 8-140
Baltimore, MD 21287

E-mail addresses:
robie@umich.edu (R. Silbergleit)
rgeocad1@jhmi.edu (R. G. Geocadin)

Rapid Focused Neurological Assessment in the Emergency Department and ICU

Joshua N. Goldstein, MD, PhD[a],*, David M. Greer, MD, MA[b]

KEYWORDS

- Neurologic examination • Physical examination
- Emergency medicine • Critical care

In the course of medical training, students learn to perform a comprehensive neurologic evaluation. A careful examination permits practitioners to discuss and pinpoint the location of a potential neuroanatomic lesion and provides clues to an underlying diagnosis. In the busy setting of an emergency department (ED) or intensive care unit (ICU), however, a detailed examination can be difficult or impractical to perform. Patients may be unconscious, intubated, hooked up to complex equipment, unstable, or otherwise unable to fully participate in the evaluation. In addition, time-sensitive diagnostic and therapeutic interventions, such as thrombolysis for acute stroke, can leave little time for the traditional comprehensive examination. The goal is to provide efficiency and focus to the evaluation, without sacrificing accuracy of diagnosis, triage, or treatment. The astute clinician working in the ED or ICU continues to keep all of the tools of the neurologic evaluation available, but applies the necessary tools at the correct times to provide a rapid and accurate diagnosis.

FOCAL COMPLAINTS

Examples of focal complaints include difficulties with speech, vision, power, sensation, or balance/coordination. A careful history should include multiple elements, including the time course of the presentation, the constellation of presenting symptoms, events

Dr. Goldstein has received consulting fees from Novo Nordisk, CSL Behring, and Genetech.
Dr. Greer has served on the speakers' bureau for Boehringer-Ingelheim Pharmaceuticals, Inc.
[a] Department of Emergency Medicine, Massachusetts General Hospital, Zero Emerson Place, Suite 3B, Boston, MA 02114, USA
[b] Department of Neurology, Massachusetts General Hospital, ACC 739A, MGH, 55 Fruit Street, Boston, MA 02114, USA
* Corresponding author.
E-mail address: jgoldstein@partners.org (J.N. Goldstein).

Emerg Med Clin N Am 27 (2009) 1–16
doi:10.1016/j.emc.2008.07.002
0733-8627/08/$ – see front matter © 2009 Elsevier Inc. All rights reserved.

emed.theclinics.com

surrounding the onset of symptoms, recent and prior medical illnesses, and the use of medications, alcohol, tobacco, or illicit drugs. The brain is an organ with specific localization of function, and the clinician should be mindful while taking the history to recognize the company that an affected brain area keeps. For example, in a patient presenting with right arm weakness, it is useful to probe for any speech/language difficulties that might suggest a lesion in the left hemisphere in the middle cerebral artery territory.

The time course of the presenting illness should be elucidated: focal symptoms with a sudden onset should always suggest stroke, either ischemic or hemorrhagic, and should trigger the clinician to begin setting the wheels in motion for an urgent evaluation (including laboratory tests and neuroimaging) as early as possible. This urgency helps to prevent delays in treatment, such as intravenous thrombolysis, which is currently approved by the US Food and Drug Administration for ischemic stroke within a 3-hour time window.[1] Multiple studies have shown a much stronger benefit for patients treated earlier within this time window,[2,3] highlighting the need for rapid treatment. There are multiple exclusion criteria (**Box 1**),[4] and clinicians who believe they have more time to evaluate the patient before treatment often take longer,[5] potentially obviating the benefit of early treatment. Symptoms with a more gradual onset may be reflective of a stroke in evolution, but more often indicate a more subacute process, such as demyelination, migraine, or neoplasm.

A rapid history should also include a history of the surrounding events. What was the patient doing when the symptoms began? Did the symptoms fluctuate? Were they maximal at onset? Had there been any recent trauma, illness, or medication changes? Has the patient ever experienced symptoms like these before? Are there any associated symptoms, including headache, chest pain, shortness of breath? What is the relevant past medical history, including medication use? Alcohol, tobacco, and drug use history should also be quickly elicited, and if the patient or family is not able to provide this history, an alcohol level and toxicology panel should be obtained.

In the ED and ICU the first order of business is securing hemodynamic and respiratory functions; however, a focused neurologic examination should then be undertaken as soon as feasible. Some patients may require urgent intubation for respiratory dysfunction or airway protection. The clinician should recognize, however, that once intubated the patient's neurologic examination is greatly limited, and thus even a cursory evaluation of language function or note of asymmetric motor activity before pharmacologic paralysis and intubation may be extremely informative. This examination serves an important baseline, which can help define the acute course of action (ie, diagnostic and therapeutic options) and prognosis. Outside of a "crash" airway, even an urgent intubation requires appropriate airway assessment, preparation, and preoxygenation,[6] and a rapid examination can be performed during this time. The clinician should focus the examination according to the area of chief complaint, and for other findings that would be expected for a lesion in the same anatomic distribution. For patients in whom a diagnosis of stroke is being entertained, a National Institutes of Health Stroke Scale can be performed within minutes to give a rapid and standardized assessment of the stroke and its severity (**Table 1**).[7,8]

The cerebral circulation can be separated into anterior and posterior circulations (**Fig. 1**).[9] The anterior circulation stems from the internal carotid arteries (ICA), which subsequently give rise to the ophthalmic, anterior choroidal, middle cerebral (MCA), and anterior cerebral arteries (ACA), and their subsequent branches. Collateral circulation across the circle of Willis is provided from both the contralateral internal carotid artery (by way of the anterior communicating artery) and the posterior circulation. The circle of Willis is incomplete in 60% of the population.[10] The posterior circulation originates in the vertebral arteries, one of which is typically dominant to the other, joining to

---

Box 1
American Stroke Association inclusion criteria for use of intravenous recombinant tissue plasminogen activator

Diagnosis of ischemic stroke causing measurable neurologic deficit.

The neurologic signs should not be clearing spontaneously.

The neurologic signs should not be minor and isolated.

Caution should be exercised in treating a patient who has major deficits.

The symptoms of stroke should not be suggestive of subarachnoid hemorrhage.

Onset of symptoms <3 hours before beginning treatment.

No head trauma or prior stroke in the previous 3 months.

No myocardial infarction in the previous 3 months.

No gastrointestinal or urinary tract hemorrhage in previous 21 days.

No major surgery in the previous 14 days.

No arterial puncture at a noncompressible site in the previous 7 days.

No history of previous intracranial hemorrhage.

Blood pressure not elevated (systolic <185 mm Hg and diastolic <110 mm Hg).

No evidence of active bleeding or acute trauma (fracture) on examination.

Not taking an oral anticoagulant or, if anticoagulant being taken, INR ≤1.7.

If receiving heparin in previous 48 hours, aPTT must be in normal range.

Platelet count ≥100,000/μL.

Blood glucose concentration ≥50 mg/dL (2.7 mmol/L).

No seizure with postictal residual neurologic impairments.

CT does not show a multilobar infarction (hypodensity >1/3 cerebral hemisphere).

The patient or family members understand the potential risks and benefits from treatment.

Data from Adams HP Jr, del Zoppo G, Alberts MJ, et al. Guidelines for the early management of adults with ischemic stroke: a guideline from the American heart association/American stroke association stroke council, clinical cardiology council, cardiovascular radiology and intervention council, and the atherosclerotic peripheral vascular disease and quality of care outcomes in research interdisciplinary working groups: the American academy of neurology affirms the value of this guideline as an educational tool for neurologists. Stroke 2007;38:1655.

---

form the basilar artery, which gives off numerous small penetrating vessels to the brainstem before bifurcating to form the two posterior cerebral arteries (PCAs). The posterior communicating arteries originate from the PCAs, completing the circle of Willis. Sometimes a PCA may originate from the ipsilateral ICA, the so-called "fetal variant PCA".[11,12]

The following is a review of common stroke symptoms that suggest a vascular distribution to the complaints (also in **Table 2**). It has been suggested that the findings that best differentiate a stroke include facial paresis, arm drift, and abnormal speech.[13]

Language Difficulties

Language difficulties should be separated into aphasias and dysarthrias, although sometimes it may be hard to distinguish in a patient who complains of difficulty "getting the words out right." It is important to decipher whether the patient means that the words were "slurred" or that they could not make the correct words. Were they having trouble

Table 1
National Institutes of Health Stroke Scale score

1a. Level of consciousness	0 = Alert; keenly responsive 1 = Not alert, but arousable by minor stimulation 2 = Not alert; requires repeated stimulation 3 = Unresponsive or responds only with reflex
1b. Level of consciousness questions:	0 = Both answers correct
What is the month? What is your age? 1c. Level of consciousness commands:	1 = Answers one question correctly 2 = Answers two questions correctly 0 = Performs both tasks correctly
Open and close your eyes. Grip and release your hand.	1 = Performs one task correctly 2 = Performs neither task correctly
2. Best gaze	0 = Normal 1 = Partial gaze palsy 2 = Forced deviation
3. Visual	0 = No visual loss 1 = Partial hemianopia 2 = Complete hemianopia 3 = Bilateral hemianopia
4. Facial palsy	0 = Normal symmetric movements 1 = Minor paralysis 2 = Partial paralysis 3 = Complete paralysis of one or both sides

5. Motor arm
  5a. Left arm
  5b. Right arm
	0 = No drift
	1 = Drift
	2 = Some effort against gravity
	3 = No effort against gravity; limb falls
	4 = No movement

6. Motor leg
  6a. Left leg
  6b. Right leg
	0 = No drift
	1 = Drift
	2 = Some effort against gravity
	3 = No effort against gravity
	4 = No movement

7. Limb ataxia	0 = Absent 1 = Present in one limb 2 = Present in two limbs
8. Sensory	0 = Normal; no sensory loss 1 = Mild-to-moderate sensory loss 2 = Severe to total sensory loss
9. Best language	0 = No aphasia; normal 1 = Mild to moderate aphasia 2 = Severe aphasia 3 = Mute, global aphasia
10. Dysarthria	0 = Normal 1 = Mild to moderate dysarthria 2 = Severe dysarthria
11. Extinction and inattention	0 = No abnormality 1 = Visual, tactile, auditory, spatial, or personal inattention 2 = Profound hemi-inattention or extinction

Total score = 0–42.

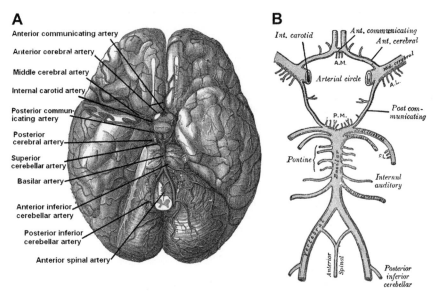

Fig. 1. Circle of Willis. (*A*) Cerebral vasculature. (*B*) Diagram of cerebral vasculature (*Reprinted from* Gray H. Anatomy of the human body. 20th edition. Philadelphia: Lea & Febinger; 1918.)

thinking of the right word to say? Were they having trouble understanding what was being said by others? Were they making frequent paraphasic errors in their speech?

Dysarthria is commonly thought of as a symptom of a posterior circulation stroke, but it can be caused by a lesion affecting any part of the speech system, including the palate, tongue, or lips/face. For example, patients who have a VIIth nerve palsy may have facial weakness causing dysarthric speech. Lesions affecting tongue or palate movement, however, are more suggestive of a brainstem lesion, and the clinician should focus the history toward symptoms/signs otherwise involving the posterior circulation. A useful bedside tool to test the location of dysfunction in dysarthric speech is to test each location of the speech mechanics separately: have the patient say "pa pa pa" to test labial function, "ta ta ta" to test lingual function, and "ka ka ka" to test palatal function. Finally, have the patient say "Pawtucket Pawtucket Pawtucket" to hear all three in comparison to one another.

Aphasias can be thought of as primarily expressive or receptive, but sometimes are mixed. The handedness of the patient is helpful in localization, because the vast majority of right-handed people have language in the left hemisphere, and around 20% to 30% of left-handed people have language in the right hemisphere. An expressive aphasia is suggestive of a lesion in the distribution of the anterior/superior division of the MCA, and a receptive aphasia is suggestive of the inferior/posterior division.

Vision Difficulties

Vision difficulties include vision loss and diplopia. Vision loss should be classified as monocular or binocular. Monocular vision loss that comes on suddenly and painlessly is most commonly vascular in origin. Because the ophthalmic artery is the first intracranial branch of the ICA, one must urgently evaluate for carotid stenosis, because transient monocular blindness may be the harbinger of a major hemispheric stroke. Binocular vision loss occurs from lesions posterior to the optic chiasm, and the

Table 2 Partial list of major stroke syndromes	
Carotid	Aphasia (dominant hemisphere) or neglect (nondominant hemisphere) Contralateral homonymous hemianopsia Contralateral motor/sensory loss of face, arm, and leg Conjugate ipsilateral eye deviation
MCA	Aphasia (dominant hemisphere) or neglect (nondominant hemisphere) Contralateral homonymous hemianopsia Contralateral motor/sensory loss face/arm > leg
ACA	Apathy, abulia, disinhibition Conjugate eye deviation Contralateral motor/sensory loss leg > arm
PICA	Ipsilateral palatal weakness, Horner syndrome Wallenberg syndrome Ipsilateral limb ataxia Decreased pain/temperature contralateral body
AICA	Ipsilateral deafness Ipsilateral facial motor/sensory loss Ipsilateral limb ataxia Decreased pain/temperature contralateral body
Basilar	Altered consciousness Oculomotor difficulties, facial paresis Ataxia, quadriparesis

Abbreviations: ACA, anterior cerebral artery; AICA, anterior inferior cerebellar artery; MCA, middle cerebral artery; PICA, posterior inferior cerebellar artery.
Data from Goetz CG. Textbook of clinical neurology. 3rd edition. Philadelphia: Elsevier; 2007.

most common vascular cause is an infarct in the visual pathways. Occipital strokes (PCA territory) cause congruous defects that typically do not have altitudinal predominance, but strokes affecting the temporal or parietal lobes (MCA territory) may cause a superior or inferior quadrantanopia, respectively.

Weakness

Weakness can affect the face or extremities. When the face only is affected, the examination is focused on differentiating a peripheral from central lesion (usually the forehead is involved in a peripheral lesion, from the level of the nucleus cranial nerve and distally, but is spared with lesions involving regions rostral to the cranial nerve nucleus). For the extremities, face and arm greater than leg weakness may suggest a lesion involving the superior division of the MCA territory, whereas isolated or primary leg weakness suggests an ACA territory lesion. Subcortical lesions commonly cause more proximal than distal weakness ("person-in-the-barrel syndrome"), whereas smaller more distal cortical lesions can cause focal weakness, such as isolated hand palsy. A patient who has profound weakness of the face, arm, and leg does not necessarily have a large stroke; in fact, if there are few other hemispheric signs (such as eye deviation, neglect, or aphasia), the lesion is most likely a small subcortical lacune in the posterior limb of the internal capsule, subcortical white matter, or even the pons.

Sensory

Sensory lesions are often difficult to characterize anatomically, and when detected are often helpful mostly when seen in conjunction with weakness for localization. Pain, rather than simply sensory loss, is more likely attributable to a peripheral cause, such as a radicular lesion.

Balance/Coordination

Balance/coordination should be tested in the limbs and axially. Common tests for cerebellar function include the finger-nose-finger and heel-knee-shin tests. The clinician must always test gait, especially when a patient presents with acute onset of dizziness. A lesion in the medial cerebellum may cause minimal impact on the bedside examination, but the patient may have profound difficulty walking, especially with tandem gait. In patients who are nonambulatory at baseline, midline cerebellar function may be tested by having them sit on the edge of a bed, attempting to steady themselves without the use of their hands or feet.

The "dizzy" patient is a common clinical conundrum in the ED, and the evaluation is covered in detail in another article in this issue. "Dizzy" may be lightheadedness to some and vertigo to others, and it is not clear that patients can reliably describe or categorize the quality of their dizziness.[14] This problem highlights the importance of a focused neurologic examination evaluating the posterior circulation and brainstem territories. Abnormalities in gait, rapid alternating movements, visual fields, and extraocular movements may not be apparent unless explicitly tested.

Patients Unable to Actively Participate in the Examination

It is important to recall when testing focal deficits that there are certain elements of the examination that can always be performed rapidly and reliably, even in uncooperative patients. These include cranial nerve reflexes (such as the pupillary and corneal reflexes), deep tendon reflexes, and pathologic reflexes (such as the Babinski sign). These tests may be performed routinely and in a minimal amount of time, and can be invaluable in determining whether an upper motor neuron lesion is present (particularly useful in suspected cases of psychogenic presentations).

GLOBAL COMPLAINTS: HEAD INJURY, SEIZURE, HEADACHE
Head Injury

The initial evaluation of any patient who has a head injury includes not only the ABCs (airway, breathing, circulation) but also securing the cervical spine during the evaluation. Patients who have head injury are at high risk for concomitant injuries to the cervical spine, and should be placed in a hard cervical collar until an unstable bony or ligamentous injury is ruled out.

The examination should be done rapidly, and following the ABCs the level of consciousness should be assessed, followed by cranial nerve function, movement in the extremities, and sensation, particularly evaluating for a sensory level in suspected spinal cord injury. The Glasgow Coma Scale is a widely used scoring system for evaluating injury severity (**Table 3**).[15,16] In general, a patient who has any new neurologic abnormality (or altered level of consciousness) following head injury should receive an emergency noncontrast head CT.[17] Such patients are also typically candidates for radiographic examination of the cervical spine,[18] and a cervical spine fracture with neurologic abnormality can be evaluated with noncontrast CT of the cervical spine and CT angiography of the head and neck to evaluate for carotid or vertebral dissection.[19]

Seizures

Seizures are classified as generalized or partial. Generalized seizures involve both hemispheres and lead to loss of consciousness. Partial seizures involve only part of the brain and can be simple or complex, with the distinction that complex partial

Table 3 Glasgow Coma Scale score	
Best eye response	1. No eye opening 2. Eye opening to pain 3. Eye opening to verbal command 4. Eyes open spontaneously
Best verbal response[a]	1. No verbal response 2. Incomprehensible sounds 3. Inappropriate words 4. Confused 5. Oriented
Best motor response	1. No motor response 2. Extension to pain 3. Flexion to pain 4. Withdrawal from pain 5. Localizing pain 6. Obeys commands

[a] For patients who are intubated, the verbal response may be imputed from the motor and eye scores as follows:

	GCS Eye Score			
GCS Motor Score	1	2	3	4
1	1	1	1	2
2	1	2	2	2
3	2	2	3	3
4	2	3	3	4
5	3	3	4	4
6	3	4	4	5

From Meredith W, Rutledge R, Fakhry SM, et al. The conundrum of the Glasgow Coma Scale in intubated patients: a linear regression prediction of the Glasgow verbal score from the Glasgow eye and motor scores. J Trauma 1998;44:839.

seizures affect the level of consciousness and behavior. Simple partial seizures typically only affect one region of the brain and cause focal symptoms referable to that region, such as motor twitching, localized convulsions, or even aphasia. Generalized seizures may start as simple partial seizures and secondarily generalize with loss of consciousness.

The evaluation of the patient who has active seizures in the ED requires a team of personnel to perform the history and examination and initiate treatment simultaneously. The history should include the events surrounding the onset of the seizure, including whether the patient may have injured his or her head before or during the event. Recent medical illnesses should be asked about, and a medication list, especially regarding the use of antiepileptic drugs (AED), should be procured. If the patient is known to have seizures previously, then medication compliance with AED therapy should be assessed.

The examination should, again, begin with ABCs, with a low threshold for securing the airway in a patient who has been having unabated generalized seizures for more than 5 minutes. Once the cardiopulmonary system is stable, the neurologic examination should focus on any specific territory believed to be involved. The motor system may need to be tested by response to painful stimulation in each extremity. Reflex testing can be performed even in the intubated patient and can be of tremendous value. As with traumatic brain injury, the cervical spine should be protected until exonerated if injury is suspected. Continuous electroencephalographic (EEG) monitoring can be useful in chemically paralyzed, sedated, or otherwise comatose patients, and failure to improve clinically despite a lack of external signs of seizures should prompt consideration of nonconvulsive status epilepticus.[20]

Pseudoseizures

Pseudoseizures can be difficult to differentiate from seizures.[21,22] The diagnosis is often made only after video and EEG monitoring,[23] and even these can be misread.[24] Although an evaluation for nonanatomic neurologic abnormalities (as discussed later) may help, the diagnosis of pseudoseizure should be made with great care or even avoided in the acute setting.

Headache

The emergency evaluation of headache should focus on a short list of defined urgent causes, including cerebrovascular events, infectious/inflammatory processes, and mass lesions. The neurologic assessment should focus on uncovering any neurologic abnormalities that might suggest an anatomic lesion. Any new neurologic abnormality should be explained with further evaluation, including neuroimaging. The evaluation and management of headache are discussed in detail in another article in this issue.

ALTERED LEVEL OF CONSCIOUSNESS: ENCEPHALOPATHY, COMA, BRAIN DEATH
Encephalopathy

Also known as altered mental status, encephalopathy is a challenging diagnostic dilemma in the ED and ICU, and a broad differential diagnosis is critical. A careful history may quickly give clues to the underlying diagnosis. Symptoms with a sudden onset and focal deficits should suggest a vascular cause (see previous section on focal deficits), either ischemic or hemorrhagic. Seizures do not necessarily present with overt clinical motor manifestations; sometimes, unusual behavior or a depressed level of consciousness may be the only sign. Metabolic abnormalities commonly cause altered mental status, particularly alterations in sodium and glucose, and hypomagnesemia should be considered as a precipitant in patients prone to seizures. Hyperammonemia and uremia should be considered in the proper clinical context. Medications commonly cause alterations in mental status, and a careful medication history should be sought, including the use of alcohol and illicit drugs. As a general rule, older patients are more sensitive to medication side effects. Tumors and other mass lesions typically arise with a more insidious onset, perhaps simply causing progressive headache and personality changes with growth over time in areas such as the frontal, temporal, or parietal lobes. An acute presentation can occur with hemorrhage into a brain neoplasm, however, or with acute brain metastases. The presence of fever or an elevated white blood cell count should alert the physician to the possibility of infection, and bacterial, viral, or fungal infections may affect the central nervous system. Meningitis with an intense inflammatory reaction may cause meningeal signs, and focal symptoms should signal the possibility of a focal cerebritis or abscess formation. Some viral infections, such as herpes simplex, have a predilection for the temporal lobes and may cause seizures early in their course. The neurologic examination may be limited because these patients may be unable to cooperate; however, testing for reflexes and response to painful stimulation can always be performed and may help localize a lesion.

Coma

Coma may be considered the far end of the spectrum for many of the disorders that cause encephalopathy. It is strictly defined as a state in which there is no awareness of the self or the environment, from which the patient cannot be aroused. In the comatose state, brainstem reflexes may be present (**Box 2**), along with reflexive response without meaningful intent, such as eye opening, grimacing, withdrawal to pain, or posturing. Patients in coma represent a medical emergency; the clinician must respond to this state quickly, ensuring protection of the airway and circulation, while concomitantly working the patient up rapidly for an underlying cause. In most cases, the longer the patient remains in the comatose state the less likely he or she will reach a level of good recovery.

Brain Death

Brain death is a state in which there is irreversible cessation of function of the entire brain, including the brainstem. Specific criteria for the diagnosis and documentation of brain death are generally defined at a local or institutional level, but several general principles described here are usually incorporated. The underlying cause of the neurologic state should be known, and it should be known to be irreversible. There must be no confounding factors to the coma examination, including hypothermia, drug intoxication, or severe metabolic, acid–base, or endocrine disorders. The patient who is brain dead must be in coma and have no preserved brainstem reflexes whatsoever. The patient must be apneic, which is tested in a formal manner (**Box 3**). Brain death is generally determined by clinical examination, often repeated at specified intervals, but if certain aspects of the clinical examination cannot be performed or are drawn into question, ancillary testing must be performed to support the diagnosis of brain death. This testing may include conventional cerebral angiography, electroencephalography, single photon emission CT, and transcranial Doppler. Brain death is a legal definition of death, and the diagnosis is rarely made in the acute setting because it requires

---

Box 2
Brainstem reflexes in the comatose patient

Pupils: Evaluate direct and consensual pupillary constriction.

Oculocephalic: Turn head side to side. Eyes should move conjugately in opposite direction of head movement.

Oculovestibular: Elevate head of bed to 30°. Clear the canal of cerumen/blood, and ensure integrity of the tympanic membrane. Irrigate the external auditory canal with ice cold water for 60 seconds. There should be tonic deviation of the eyes toward the cold irrigated ear, with fast component nystagmus in the opposite direction.

Grimace: Insert a Q-tip in to the nostril; observe for facial movement. Apply pressure to the supraorbital ridge or temporomandibular joint.

Corneal reflex: Stimulation of cornea should trigger eyelid closure.

Gag reflex: Stimulation of the soft palate should cause symmetric elevation. Stimulation of the pharyngeal mucosa should cause the patient to gag (this is often evaluated incidentally during airway evaluation and management).

Extremities: Noxious stimulation may be applied to the nail bed of the fingers or toes. Extensor posturing involves movement toward the noxious stimulus. Flexor posturing may be more difficult to distinguish; stereotyped flexor movement regardless of where the noxious stimulus is applied is consisted with pathologic posturing.

Box 3
Apnea testing

The patient should be hemodynamically stable, off of vasopressor medications.

Preoxygenate the patient with 100% F_{IO_2} for 30 minutes before testing.

Adjust the ventilator to achieve a normal pH (7.35–7.45) and normocarbia (35–45 mm Hg, or within 5 mm of the patient's baseline if a known CO_2 retainer).

Disconnect the ventilator and supply a continuous oxygen source by way of the endotracheal tube.

Observe the patient for chest or abdominal wall movement, cyanosis, hypoxia, or hemodynamic instability, all of which should trigger termination of the test. At no point should the patient become hypoxic during apnea testing.

After 8 to 10 minutes, draw an arterial blood gas and reconnect the ventilator

The apnea test is positive if the P_{CO_2} increases above 60 mm Hg, or 20 mm above the baseline.

If the test was indeterminate, but the patient was stable during testing, it may be repeated for a longer time interval to achieve the necessary parameters.

---

a comprehensive workup for treatable causes. The local organ procurement officer should be contacted for the possibility of organ donation in cases of brain death or other neurologic catastrophes when there is no chance of neurologic recovery.

NECK / BACK PAIN

A careful history helps elucidate the level of neurologic dysfunction in the patient presenting with neck or back pain. The clinician can then target the examination to help risk-stratify whether the patient requires an emergency diagnostic workup to rule out acute cord compression or cauda equina syndrome. The nature of any injury is highly important, and for patients either "found down" or with a suspected flexion or extension injury a cervical collar should be placed for stabilization. Useful symptoms to inquire about include the presence and pattern of pain, weakness, or sensation loss/dysesthesias, along with bowel or bladder difficulties and gait disturbances.

A rapid examination should include motor and sensory function, reflexes, and saddle anesthesia/rectal tone when needed. Motor weakness and sensation loss may fit into any of several patterns, depending on the level of impairment, ranging from the cord to the distal peripheral nerve. A sensory level on the torso may indicate a level of cord impingement/dysfunction. For patients who have bowel or bladder complaints, perianal sensation and rectal tone should be tested. Bladder function can be assessed by testing for postvoid residual, either with a straight catheter or bedside ultrasound.[25] The deep tendon reflexes are extremely helpful. Hyperreflexia and up-going toes are consistent with an upper motor neuron lesion. Depressed reflexes are more suggestive of a lower motor neuron process, but may be seen also with acute cord injuries. **Table 4** gives a listing of common radiculopathies.

Specific syndromes can relate from injury to specific regions of the spinal cord. Cervicomedullary syndrome occurs with a high cervical cord injury, leading to quadriparesis (typically affecting the arms greater than legs), hypoesthesia, and symptoms affecting the lower brainstem, such as perioral numbness, hypotension, and hypoventilation. Central cord syndrome causes preferential weakness in the upper extremities, but sensory loss in the upper and lower extremities. Anterior cord syndrome causes paralysis and sensory loss to pain and temperature below the level of the lesion,

Table 4
Findings in common radiculopathies

Disc	Root	Pain/Dysesthesias	Sensory Loss	Weakness	Reflex Loss
C4-5	C5	Neck, shoulder, upper arm	Shoulder	Deltoid, biceps, infraspinatus	Biceps
C5-6	C6	Neck, shoulder, lateral arm, radial forearm, thumb, index finger	Lateral arm, radial forearm, thumb, index finger	Biceps, brachioradialis, supinator	Biceps, brachioradialis
C6-7	C7	Neck, lateral arm, ring through index finger	Radial forearm, index and middle fingers	Triceps, extensor carpi ulnaris	Triceps
C7-T1	C8	Ulnar forearm and hand	Ulnar half or ring finger, little finger	Intrinsic hand muscles, wrist extensors, flexor digitorum profundus	Finger flexion
L3-4	L4	Anterior thigh, inner shin	Anteromedial thigh and shin, inner foot	Quadriceps	Patella
L4-5	L5	Lateral thigh and calf, dorsum of foot, great toe	Lateral calf and great toe	Extensor hallices longus, ± foot dorsiflexion, inversion and eversion	None
L5-S1	S1	Back of thigh, lateral posterior calf, lateral foot	Posterolateral calf, lateral and sole of foot, smaller toes	Gastrocnemius ± foot eversion	Achilles

with preserved vibratory and position sense. Brown-Séquard syndrome results from injury to half of the cord, leading to ipsilateral hemiparesis and dorsal column sensation loss, and contralateral pain and temperature loss. Cauda equina syndrome results from injury to the lumbosacral roots, causing weakness, sensory deficits, and hyporeflexia in the lower extremities, and bowel, bladder, and sexual dysfunction.

GENERALIZED WEAKNESS

The patient presenting with generalized weakness raises an initially large differential diagnosis, but one that can be honed quickly based on the history. Generalized weakness may be described by patients who are presyncopal, in metabolic disarray, intoxicated, anemic, chronically ill, or simply fatigued. A rapid neurologic examination can determine any focal findings, in which case the evaluation should be targeted as in the earlier section on focal complaints, and a diagnosis that explains these findings pursued. Although generalized weakness might be a manifestation of stroke, such as a basilar artery occlusion, this would normally be accompanied by findings such as cranial nerve abnormalities and altered consciousness. Similarly, although a high cervical cord lesion could cause generalized weakness, the history would normally include neck pain or bowel/bladder disturbances.

The clinician should be aware of three other conditions that can present with rapid generalized weakness: Guillain Barré Syndrome (GBS), myasthenia gravis, and botulism. GBS commonly presents with a rapidly ascending weakness over hours to days, and in its severe form can lead to severe quadriparesis, respiratory failure, and dysautonomia. The examination is notable for symmetric weakness, very diminished or absent deep tendon reflexes, and minimal sensory derangement, and some variants may display ocular motility abnormalities and ataxia.[26] The workup consists of lumbar puncture (typically showing elevated protein but a paucity of inflammatory cells) and electromyography (EMG) with nerve conduction studies, which may show evidence of peripheral demyelination (but can be unremarkable early in the disease).

Myasthenia gravis also typically presents with generalized weakness; common additional manifestations include extraocular movement abnormalities, ptosis, and shortness of breath. An edrophonium test may be performed in a controlled setting, such as the ED or ICU, and may help confirm the diagnosis (**Box 4**). Other helpful tests include EMG with repetitive stimulation and single-fiber EMG, and specific serum antibody testing.

Botulism presents with a symmetric, descending flaccid paralysis and prominent cranial nerve palsies, including extraocular movements, dysarthria, dysphagia, and facial weakness. The limbs typically become weak over 1 to 3 days, and complete paralysis may occur. Patients are hyporeflexic and may develop fixed dilated pupils. Ileus and urinary retention commonly occur. Patients are afebrile and have normal cognition. Respiratory failure may occur, necessitating mechanical ventilation and ICU care. Diagnosis is made by detecting botulinum toxin in the blood, stool, wound site, or suspected food. EMG and nerve conduction studies may be supportive.

NONANATOMIC COMPLAINTS

Occasionally, the practitioner is faced with distinguishing complaints that have no clear anatomic source, either before or after imaging. Often the complaints do not clearly fit a neuroanatomic pattern, but may closely resemble neurologic disorders, such as disturbances of speech, vision, sensation, power, or balance, and overt manifestations mimicking recognized disorders may occur, such as in pseudoseizures or psychogenic parkinsonism. A careful history can elucidate potential underlying

---

Box 4
Edrophonium test

Perform in a monitored setting (such as the ED or ICU). Atropine should be at the bedside in case of significant bradycardia or hypotension.

Prepare two 1-mL tuberculin syringes: one placebo injection of 1 mL normal saline, and one 10 mg of edrophonium in 1 mL of solution.

Monitor a specific muscle group (eg, ptosis or upgaze) during testing to see if there is improvement.

First administer the placebo; observe for several minutes for improvement

Next, administer a test dose of 2 mg (0.2 mL) of edrophonium and observe for several minutes.

If no improvement is noted, but the patient tolerates the test dose, another 3 mg (0.3 mL) is given. If there is still no improvement, but the patient is still tolerating the doses given, the remainder of the vial (5 mg, or 0.5 mL) is given.

Improvement should occur within 15 to 30 seconds, but is typically short-lived (minutes).

causes, such as a psychiatric history (including a personality disorder), recent life stressors, preexisting organic brain disease, or secondary gain. The following tests can help distinguish organic from psychogenic presentations.

Paralysis

Hand drop

Patients who have true paralysis are unable to keep their own hand from falling on their face when an examiner drops it from an elevated position. Care must be taken in this technique so that the patient does not injure himself or herself.

Hoover sign

Hoover sign is tested by having the patient lie supine with the examiner's hands beneath both heels. When asked to raise the paretic leg, the truly paretic patient reflexively exerts downward force on the contralateral heel, whereas the psychogenic paretic patient generally fails to push down with the "good" leg.

Other testing may simply involve movement in other directions by the nonparetic leg, and seeing if there are stabilizing movements made by the "paralyzed" leg.

Visual Disorders

Psychogenic blindness may be tested by presenting the patient with a mirror, an obscene written word, or a human face with strong emotional valence. A blink to visual threat may also be helpful.

Sensory Disorders

Sensory disturbances may be tested with a tuning fork to the forehead—a patient who has psychogenic sensation loss states difficulty feeling the vibration past the midline on the hemianesthetic side. One way to test hand numbness is to ask the patient to extend both arms with thumbs down, cross the arms, clasp their hands together, and rotate their hands inward. It becomes difficult to keep track of which finger is from which hand, so that when the examiner touches each finger to test for sensation, the patient may confuse the side that is insensate.

Again, the examiner may always fall back on reflexes. Deep tendon reflexes are involuntary and difficult to mimic. Other examples include rectal tone, anal wink, and the cremasteric reflex, which may be tested in cases of purported paraplegia with nondermatomal sensory loss. The Babinski sign, or the absence thereof, may also be useful.

SUMMARY

The emergency neurologic examination cannot be comprehensive. A comprehensive examination is not always necessary in the acute setting, however. Rather, the clinician should use the chief complaint and historical features to proactively determine the type of focused neurologic history and examination to perform, facilitating rapid triage, evaluation, and treatment.

REFERENCES

1. Tissue plasminogen activator for acute ischemic stroke. The national institute of neurological disorders and stroke rt-PA stroke study group. N Engl J Med 1995;333:1581–7.
2. Hacke W, Donnan G, Fieschi C, et al. Association of outcome with early stroke treatment: pooled analysis of ATLANTIS, ECASS, and NINDS rt-PA stroke trials. Lancet 2004;363:768–74.

3. Marler JR, Tilley BC, Lu M, et al. Early stroke treatment associated with better out-come: the NINDS rt-PA stroke study. Neurology 2000;55:1649–55.
4. Adams HP Jr, del Zoppo G, Alberts MJ, et al. Guidelines for the early manage-ment of adults with ischemic stroke: a guideline from the American heart associ-ation/American stroke association stroke council, clinical cardiology council, cardiovascular radiology and intervention council, and the atherosclerotic periph-eral vascular disease and quality of care outcomes in research interdisciplinary working groups: the American academy of neurology affirms the value of this guideline as an educational tool for neurologists. Stroke 2007;38:1655.
5. Romano JG, Muller N, Merino JG, et al. In-hospital delays to stroke thrombolysis: paradoxical effect of early arrival. Neurol Res 2007;29:664–6.
6. Walls RM. Airway. In: Marx JA, Hockberger RS, Walls RM, editors, Rosen's emer-gency medicine: concepts and clinical practice, vol 1. St. Louis (MO): Mosby; 2002. p. 2.
7. Lyden P, Raman R, Liu L, et al. NIHSS training and certification using a new digital video disk is reliable. Stroke 2005;36:2446–9.
8. Powers DW. Assessment of the stroke patient using the NIH stroke scale. Emerg Med Serv 2001;30:52–6.
9. Gray H. Anatomy of the human body. 20th edition. Philadelphia: Lea & Febinger; 1918.
10. Grainger RG, Allison D, Adam A, et al, editors. Grainger & Allison's diagnostic ra-diology: a textbook of medical imaging. 4th edition. London: Harcourt Publishers Limited; 2001.
11. van Raamt AF, Mali WP, van Laar PJ, et al. The fetal variant of the circle of Willis and its influence on the cerebral collateral circulation. Cerebrovasc Dis 2006;22: 217–24.
12. Goetz CG. Textbook of clinical neurology. 3rd edition. Philadelphia: Elsevier; 2007.
13. Goldstein LB, Simel DL. Is this patient having a stroke? J Am Med Assoc 2005; 293:2391–402.
14. Newman-Toker DE, Cannon LM, Stofferahn ME, et al. Imprecision in patient reports of dizziness symptom quality: a cross-sectional study conducted in an acute care setting. Mayo Clin Proc 2007;82:1329–40.
15. Meredith W, Rutledge R, Fakhry SM, et al. The conundrum of the Glasgow coma scale in intubated patients: a linear regression prediction of the Glasgow verbal score from the Glasgow eye and motor scores. J Trauma 1998;44:839–44.
16. Moore L, Lavoie A, Camden S, et al. Statistical validation of the Glasgow Coma Score. J Trauma 2006;60:1238–43.
17. Stiell IG, Clement CM, Rowe BH, et al. Comparison of the Canadian CT head rule and the New Orleans criteria in patients with minor head injury. J Am Med Assoc 2005;294:1511–8.
18. Stiell IG, Clement CM, McKnight RD, et al. The Canadian C-spine rule versus the NEXUS low-risk criteria in patients with trauma. N Engl J Med 2003;349:2510–8.
19. Cothren CC, Moore EE, Ray CE Jr, et al. Cervical spine fracture patterns mandat-ing screening to rule out blunt cerebrovascular injury. Surgery 2007;141:76–82.
20. Towne AR, Waterhouse EJ, Boggs JG, et al. Prevalence of nonconvulsive status epilepticus in comatose patients. Neurology 2000;54:340–5.
21. Benbadis SR. How many patients with pseudoseizures receive antiepileptic drugs prior to diagnosis? Eur Neurol 1999;41:114–5.
22. Sackellares DK, Sackellares JC. Impaired motor function in patients with psycho-genic pseudoseizures. Epilepsia 2001;42:1600–6.

23. Benbadis SR, Agrawal V, Tatum WO. How many patients with psychogenic non-epileptic seizures also have epilepsy? Neurology 2001;57:915–7.
24. Benbadis SR, Tatum WO. Overinterpretation of EEGs and misdiagnosis of epilepsy. J Clin Neurophysiol 2003;20:42–4.
25. Chan H. Noninvasive bladder volume measurement. J Neurosci Nurs 1993;25:309–12.
26. Koeppen S, Kraywinkel K, Wessendorf TE, et al. Long-term outcome of Guillain-Barré syndrome. Neurocrit Care 2006;5:235–42.

Critical Care Transport of Patients Who Have Acute Neurological Emergencies

Bradley Uren, MD*, Mark J. Lowell, MD, Robert Silbergleit, MD

KEYWORDS

- Transport • Critical care • Ambulance • Helicopter
- Stroke • Brain injury

Optimal treatment of patients who have neurological emergencies often requires specialty care available only at tertiary or quaternary medical centers. Experienced critical care transport teams often are needed for the safe and rapid transport of a patient who has a neurological emergency from the scene of injury or from a health care facility that cannot provide the necessary specialty care these patients need. This article reviews the special questions and issues in critical care transport related specifically to the care of patients who have neurological emergencies. It first considers potential indications for transport and reviews attempts to create a hierarchical stroke center system akin to that developed for trauma care. It then discusses therapeutic concerns relating to the transport environment and the use of specific interventions, including the effects of end-tidal CO_2 monitoring on intracranial pressure, patient outcomes after traumatic brain injury, and opportunities to initiate therapeutic hypothermia in comatose survivors of cardiac arrest during transport. Finally, the cost of critical care transport of patients who have neurological emergencies is considered.

INDICATIONS FOR CRITICAL CARE TRANSPORT OF PATIENTS WHO HAVE NEUROLOGICAL EMERGENCIES

Critical care transport is assuming an increasing role in health care because patients who have medical conditions that exceed the capabilities of the initial treating facility require timely safe and effective transport to regional referral centers. Trauma systems provide the most familiar model, and standards exist for the transport of specific patient types to preidentifed trauma centers either directly or after initial evaluation at another hospital.

Department of Emergency Medicine and Survival Flight, University of Michigan, Ann Arbor, MI, USA
* Corresponding author.
E-mail address: bguren@umich.edu (B. Uren).

Emerg Med Clin N Am 27 (2009) 17–26
doi:10.1016/j.emc.2008.09.001
0733-8627/08/$ – see front matter © 2009 Elsevier Inc. All rights reserved.

Because of newly available treatment modalities, patients who have neurological injuries have become an increasing proportion of critical care transport operations. In particular, the advent of thrombolytic therapy for the treatment of acute ischemic stroke has led to an increased demand for transport to tertiary care centers before or after treatment.

Critical care transport is efficient for the overall health care system because it allows specialized and expensive resources and expertise to remain centralized rather than replicated in less effective and redundant or underutilized specialty services. Each patient transport, however, adds expense and involves added risk to the patient (and, arguably, to the transport team). Critically ill or injured patients are, by definition, in relatively fragile condition. Because interfacility transport requires the movement of a patient from a secure emergency department or inpatient unit to the inherently less stable environment of an ambulance, the patient is subjected to additional risk even if the transport is conducted by a well-trained and well-equipped team. Emergency medical transportation, because it is performed around the clock, usually at relatively high speeds, with necessarily short response times, on an unscheduled basis, and often in unfavorable weather conditions, is itself a risky venture, whether conducted by ground-based systems or air medical services.

Therefore it is important that the potential benefit of emergent transport outweigh the risk and cost of the transfer. The appropriate indications for critical care transport of patients who have neurological emergencies are numerous. **Table 1**, although not intended to be comprehensive, summarizes many of these indications.

The appropriate mode of transportation for patients for whom transfer is indicated depends on numerous factors. These considerations include the distance and anticipated duration of transport, the stability of the patient and the urgency of the treatment to be provided at the receiving hospital, the transport expertise and resources available at the sending facility, and other situational factors. For critically ill and injured patients who have neurological emergencies, air medical transport often is appropriate. Air medical transport may be more expensive and risky than ground transport, but in most situations it is faster, and air transport teams usually are more highly trained, more experienced, and better equipped than ground transport teams. It is important to guard against overuse of air medical transport, but few data support speculations of such misuse. In their own benchmarking experience, the authors have seen the opposite, a trend over several years toward the air transport population having increasingly higher acuity scores, and being more critically ill.[1]

THE ROLE OF PREHOSPITAL AND INTERFACILITY TRANSPORT IN PATIENTS WHO HAVE SUFFERED STROKE
Time is Brain

The advent of revascularization therapies for patients who have experienced acute ischemic stroke includes Food and Drug Administration-approved treatments, such as intravenous thrombolysis with tissue plasminogen activator (tPA), and other promising therapies, such as intra-arterial approaches to clot lysis or removal, for which definitive confirmatory studies of efficacy are not yet available. Meaningful success of any type of stroke revascularization program depends on efficient integration with prehospital and interfacility emergency medical service (EMS) systems.

Intravenous tPA must be given within 180 minutes after stroke onset, with stroke onset defined as the time the patient was last seen to be normal.[2] To determine eligibility for tPA, patients who have stroke symptoms arriving in the emergency department must undergo an evaluation that includes a rapid history and examination, a CT

| Table 1 |
| Potential indications for transport of patients who have neurologic emergencies |

Diagnosis	Indication
Acute ischemic stroke	Intravenous tPA or postthrombolytic care
	Endovascular thrombolysis/mechanical clot retrieval
	Massive stroke/consideration of hemicraniectomy
	Stroke center/stroke unit care
	Neurological critical care specialization
Intracerebral hemorrhage	Surgical drainage of selected hematomas
	Neurological critical care specialization
	Intracranial pressure monitoring and treatment
	Drainage of cerebrospinal fluid
	Consideration of thrombolysis of intraventricular clots
Traumatic brain injury	Surgical drainage of extra-axial hematomas
	Neurological critical care specialization
	Intracranial pressure monitoring/drainage
	of cerebrospinal fluid
	Advanced neuroimaging (eg, diffusion tensor imaging)
Spinal cord injury	Surgical decompression and stabilization
	Specialty care in a spinal cord injury center
Comatose survivors of cardiac arrest (hypoxic ischemic encephalopathy)	Therapeutic hypothermia/endovascular cooling
	Interventional cardiology if needed
	Neurological critical care specialization if needed
Status epilepticus	Pharmacologic coma
	Continuous electroencephalograph monitoring to titrate burst suppression
	Continuous or acute electroencephalograph monitoring in the emergency department and ICU
	Neurological critical care specialization

scan of the brain, and basic blood testing. Because the benchmark time for this evaluation and determination of eligibility is 60 minutes, patients actually must present to the emergency department within 2 hours of the stroke onset to be eligible for tPA, and earlier is even better. Truly effective stroke thrombolysis depends on prehospital EMS systems capable of rapid identification of stroke patients, collection of the critical historical elements from witnesses (eg, time last seen normal), expedited transport, and prearrival notification to allow activation of an emergency department stroke treatment protocol. Because some hospitals do not have the necessary resources to provide tPA to eligible stroke patients, EMS diversion of patients to "stroke centers" often is advocated and is discussed in more detail later.

Critical care transport services, often in combination with stroke center outreach campaigns and telemedicine stroke consultation services, can help make intravenous tPA therapy available to patients presenting at some hospitals that lack the necessary resources to provide therapy on their own. Such programs often use "drip and ship" paradigms in which the therapy is initiated at a referring hospital where the patient initially presented after consultation with physicians at a receiving stroke center, followed by critical care transport to the stroke center. Alternatively, patients simply can be transported quickly within the window for revascularization therapy. Intra-arterial therapy for acute ischemic stroke generally is performed up to 6 hours after the onset of stroke symptoms, and this treatment window may be extended for certain less common types of strokes (those involving the posterior brain circulation). Intra-arterial therapy involves thrombolysis or clot removal through special endovascular techniques that require a high degree of specialization in interventional neuroradiology. Rapid critical care inter-facility transport is essential for this kind of treatment program, because such expertise is available only in a small number of tertiary medical centers. The use of helicopter-based air medical transport for intra-arterial treatment of stroke has been described, modeled, and found to be both theoretically clinically beneficial and cost effective.[3]

Stroke Centers and Emergency Medical Service Diversion

Since 2004, The Joint Commission (TJC), in collaboration with the American Heart As-sociation (AHA)/American Stroke Association (ASA), has been certifying medical cen-ters that make exceptional efforts to foster better outcomes for patients who have had stroke as "primary stroke centers." To achieve this certification, institutions must meet specific requirements and expectations based on the Brain Attack Coalition's Recom-mendations for Primary Stroke Centers as well as guidelines developed by the AHA/ASA and other evidence-based guidelines.[4] Currently there are about 500 certified pri-mary stroke centers in the United States. A subsequent process to identify an even higher level of expertise in stroke care in facilities that would be designated "compre-hensive stroke centers" is under development.

Since the early 1990s there have been calls for ambulance diversion to self-designated stroke centers, leading to controversy and politically charged debates about EMS policy. Even when implemented, such triage efforts often were hampered or defeated simply by every hospital in a region designating itself a stroke center. The development of the TJC independent certification process has renewed these policy debates. Although such debates often focus on improving access to revascularization with tPA, this issue is only one part of the justification for diversion. It has been shown that primary stroke center certification is associated with increased use of tPA in eli-gible stroke patients,[5] but most of the performance indicators tracked for stroke cen-ter certification actually relate to inpatient rather than emergency department care. Inpatient care on a stroke unit is strongly associated with better clinical outcomes than seen with standard inpatient care. Such improvements seem to be multifactorial and multidisciplinary. Rigorous attention to blood pressure, oxygenation, and evolu-tion of neurological status help prevent secondary brain injury after stroke. In critically ill victims of stroke, access to specialists in neurocritical care and to neurosurgical options such as decompressive hemicraniectomy may offer further benefit. Prevention of systemic complications by the careful application of "low tech" care, such as enforcing swallowing precautions, deep-vein thrombosis prophylaxis, and early dis-continuation of urinary catheters, also may be important. More stringent secondary stroke-prevention efforts may be a factor also. Although there are few data available demonstrating the specific benefit of either prehospital diversion or interfacility trans-port of patients who have suffered a stroke, many find the indirect evidence compel-ling. With independent certification now being performed by the TJC, EMS systems have an opportunity to revisit and implement previously challenging diversion policies for patients who have had acute stroke.

Transportation to the nearest stroke center should be tailored to the needs of the patient. In general there are two main reasons to use critical care transport teams: the provision of advanced care, and speed of transport. The critically ill patient requires advanced therapies that ordinary interhospital crews are not trained or expe-rienced enough to provide (eg, airway and ventilator management and techniques for recognizing and treating signs of increased intracranial pressure). Depending on the distance to be traveled, speed can become important in the delivery of time-sensitive therapies; obviously, the use of rotor or fixed wing transport can help shorten the time to definitive care.

SITUATIONS AND INTERVENTIONS SPECIAL TO THE TRANSPORT OF PATIENTS WHO HAVE NEUROLOGICAL EMERGENCIES

The care provided during transport of patients who have critical neurological problems is an extension of the continuum of resuscitative efforts begun in the emergency department and continued in the ICU. This section focuses on some of the most important elements of supportive care in patients experiencing a neurological emergency, the potentially special role of careful control of ventilation in transported patients who have traumatic brain injury, and the potential opportunity for expediting the cooling of comatose survivors of cardiac arrest.

Supportive Care and the Transport Environment

Supportive care for patients who have neurological emergencies is similar in most respects to the care of other critically ill and injured patients, but some interactions between the characteristics of these patients and the transport environment deserve special attention.

The transport environment inherently subjects patients to translational and vibrational forces of unclear clinical significance. In the past, it was avoiding excessive stimulation of patients who had intracerebral or subarachnoid hemorrhage was thought to be important to reduce risk of rebleeding. Although the practice of keeping these patients in dimly lit, quiet environments is now a relic of the past, lingering concerns occasionally arise that critical care transport by ground ambulance or especially by helicopter may be particularly stimulating. Although few data are available to address this issue specifically, retrospective reviews do not corroborate this concern.[6] Furthermore, although the nature of the forces involved in patient transport differ between ground and helicopter ambulances, the energy conveyed to the patient in the two means of transport is similar.[7] Although the stimulation and movement of patients does not seem to be clinically problematic, some degree of sedation for transport is often indicated.

Sedation and paralysis often are used in the transport of critically ill or injured patients but should be used more selectively and cautiously in patients who have acute neurological emergencies. Documentation of the neurological examination in these patients is very critical before the initiation of sedation and pharmacologic paralysis. Similarly, on arrival at the tertiary receiving hospital, a follow-up neurological examination is a key factor in determining the next step in the patient's care. A change from baseline (possibly resulting from presedation and pharmacologic paralysis) to the posttransport neurological function often directs the course and aggressiveness of care. If a patient cannot be evaluated because of persistent deep sedation or long-acting paralysis, the need for life-saving interventions may not be apparent, and treatment may be delayed. Nevertheless, sedation and paralysis still should be used in the transport of patients who have neurological injury when needed for patient comfort, to provide adequate immobilization, or otherwise to ensure the safety of transport. Pharmacologic agents used for this purpose should be selected carefully, and the amounts given should be titrated to ensure the lowest effective dose is given. Ideal agents are those with short durations of action and predictable rapid recovery. Propofol is a good choice for sedation and may be titrated more easily than benzodiazepines. If benzodiazepines are needed, midazolam has a shorter duration of sedation than lorazepam or diazepam. For analgesia, ultrashort-acting narcotics such as fentanyl are preferable to morphine or hydromorphone. Among the widely available choices for nondepolarizing neuromuscular blockade, atracurium has the shortest duration of action, followed by vecuronium. Cisatracurium is longer acting, and pancuronium is much longer acting, so these agents are less preferred for the transportation of patients who have neurological emergencies. Also of relevance for transport systems is that some benzodiazepines (lorazepam) and neuromuscular blockers (atracurium/cisatracurium) call for refrigerated storage, which may be inconvenient in the transport environment.

It is important that critical care transport teams be familiar with the elements of supportive care that are especially important in patients who have neurological emergencies. These elements are not unique to the transport environment and are not discussed in detail here but are listed here because they are important for transport crews to review.

It is important to avoid hypoxia, because the injured brain may be particularly susceptible to even moderate drops in hemoglobin oxygen saturation. Continuous oxygen saturation monitoring generally is appropriate, and supplemental oxygenation should be used when needed. Another potential concern with hypoxia is the vasodilatory response, which may exacerbate intracranial pressure and worsen ongoing neurological injury.

Optimal blood pressure management in patients who have neurological emergencies is controversial. Both high and low extremes are associated with worse outcomes. Hypotension, however, is generally a more serious condition than hypertension. Permissive hypertension may be reasonable in many patients, rather than risking rapid iatrogenic decreases in the transport environment. When antihypertensives are needed, one should consider rapid-acting beta-blockers (labetalol) or cerebral circulation–selective calcium-channel blockers (nicardipine). Nitrate vasodilators (eg, nitroprusside) also can be used acutely, but their sustained use has been associated with increased intracranial pressure, and therefore these agents have fallen out of favor in neurocritical care.

Hyperthermia exacerbates acute brain injury and should be avoided. Antipyretics are important to treat elevated temperatures because of fever, and environmental conditions such as ambient temperature and bundling of the patient should be controlled to prevent situational hyperthermia. Intravenous fluid warmers or blood warmers and heated ventilator circuits, even though rarely used in the transport environment, should not be used in hyperthermic patients who have neurological emergencies. In these situations the therapeutic target is normothermia, with the exception of therapeutic hypothermia in patients who have experienced cardiac arrest, as discussed later.

Interventions that may be required for a patient after a neurological insult fall within the scope of practice of most critical care transport providers. The crew configuration of critical care transport services is variable, however, ranging from a physician/nurse team to a paramedic/respiratory therapist team. The scope of practice therefore can differ widely between crews, and it behooves the transferring physician to be familiar with and understand these differences so the appropriate crew is used.

Use of End-Tidal CO₂ Monitoring in the Transport of Patients Who Have Traumatic Brain Injury

Cerebral autoregulation and CO_2 reactivity are key determinants of cerebral blood flow and can affect outcome after brain injury. Both hypoventilation and hyperventilation pose risks. Hypoventilation resulting in elevated partial pressure of carbon dioxide (pCO_2) causes cerebrovascular dilatation and increased intracranial pressures. Elevated intracranial pressure reduces cerebral perfusion pressure and can reduce cerebral blood flow, causing secondary ischemic injury. Uncontrolled elevated intra-cranial pressure also can cause further secondary mechanical brain injury and ulti-mately can result in brain herniation syndromes. Hyperventilation, on the other hand, reduces pCO_2 and causes cerebrovascular vasoconstriction, which can reduce intracranial pressure. Excessive or prolonged hyperventilation, however, leads to re-duction in cerebral blood flow sufficient to cause secondary ischemic injury and poor outcome. Current recommendations are to provide "normal ventilatory rates" in patients who have moderate to severe brain injury to maintain end-tidal CO_2 ($ETCO_2$) levels of 35 to 40 mm Hg.

Patients who have moderate to severe traumatic brain injury often are obtunded or comatose. They are at risk of both hypoventilation and elevated intracranial pressure from the primary injury. Theoretically, therefore, early endotracheal intubation and as-sisted ventilation are important therapeutic interventions in these patients. Actual clin-ical experience with early intubation and ventilation of patients who have suffered traumatic brain injury before transport to a tertiary care facility has been mixed, prob-ably because of frequent overventilation.

It has been common in the training of many medical and paramedical providers to emphasize the value of hyperventilation in forestalling brain herniation and to explain inadequately the risks of ventilating too much. Furthermore, it has been shown that hyper-ventilation by a bag-valve device is a common psychomotor error even in well-trained medical personnel in emergency situations after successful endotracheal intubation. In short, it is common for transport teams to overuse hyperventilation, either because they think it is necessary or because it is easy to do inadvertently. Feedback devices have been shown reduce the use of hyperventilation. End-tidal capnometry now is avail-able in the transport environment to help guide adequacy of ventilation.

Evidence supporting the use of $ETCO_2$ monitoring in the transport of patients who have traumatic brain injury comes from the work of Davis and colleagues[8,9] in the San Diego Paramedic Rapid Sequence Intubation Trial and subsequent analyses. This study showed that patients who had traumatic brain injury undergoing rapid-sequence intuba-tion did less well than historical controls before adoption of paramedic rapid-sequence intubation. Secondary analyses of that trial and of the larger San Diego trauma registry suggested that hyperventilation and hypocapnia are the major contributors to adverse outcomes and mortality in patients who have traumatic brain injury after adjusting for multiple other covariates. Ground crews in San Diego were not equipped with $ETCO_2$ equipment. Interestingly, patients who had traumatic brain injury who were intubated and transported by air medical crews, all of whom were equipped with $ETCO_2$ monitoring, had improved outcomes not attributable to any other covariate.[10]

Transport ventilators and $ETCO_2$ monitoring now are used by many transport services and allow consistent titrateable ventilation. These devices can use sidestream or mainstream monitoring technologies, both of which work well in adults at normal respiratory rates. In the absence of definitive prospective clinical trial data, the available evidence supports the routine use of these devices in patients who have traumatic brain injury and suggests their use directly improves patient outcomes.[11,12] Less evidence is available for the use of this technology in the transport of patients who have other neurological emergencies, but, given the similarities in the underlying pathophysiology, it is easy to extrapolate that $ETCO_2$ may be useful after other forms of brain injury as well.

Expedited Initiation of Therapeutic Hypothermia During Transport

Therapeutic cooling of comatose survivors of cardiac arrest to 32°C to 34°C within hours after the return of spontaneous circulation has been shown in two randomized clinical trials to improve the proportion of patients who have favorable neurological outcomes.[13,14] The use of therapeutic hypothermia now is recommended in the Emergency Cardiac Care Guidelines of the AHA for selected victims of out-of-hospital cardiac arrest. Use of the therapy has been gaining momentum slowly in medical centers in the United States. At present, the experience and technologies to provide this therapy still are concentrated in a limited number of institutions, but wider adoption is projected to have a substantial public health impact.[15] The use of critical care transport to make this therapy available to comatose survivors initially taken to hospitals without this capability by taking them to centers with this capability is promising but nascent. The use of this therapy by critical care transport teams offers a potential opportunity to initiate cooling before arrival at the receiving facility. There are no established clinical data with which to determine how quickly patients should be cooled after global cerebral ischemia, but it generally is recommended that cooling be initiated as early as possible. Some degree of cooling may be accomplished simply by having transport teams avoid the interventions used to prevent environmental cooling described earlier: warmed blankets, warmed fluids, and heated ventilator circuits. A variety of both low-tech and high-tech methods for initiating and maintaining hypothermia exist, but many of the definitive cooling strategies begun in the emergency department and continued in the ICU are not amenable to the critical care transport environment. Some, like the use of water baths, are not practical. Others, like endovascular cooling or the use of advanced surface cooling devices, require large and heavy bedside cooling consoles.

Recent experience suggests that iced saline infusions stand out as the best candidate method for initiating cooling during transport. The rapid infusion over 30 to 60 minutes of 2 to 4 L of refrigerated normal saline at 4°C has been shown to reduce core body temperature by 1.5°C to 4°C in comatose survivors of cardiac arrest.[16-20] In several safety studies, this method of cooling was not associated with adverse consequences in terms of blood pressure, heart rate, arterial oxygenation, evidence of pulmonary edema on initial chest radiograph, or re-arrest. This technique is more effective than would be expected if temperature change occurred evenly through all parts of the body, suggesting that temperature can be considered to have a volume of distribution. Initially, cold saline infusions seem to cool the core selectively. Although cold saline infusions do not seem to be an effective strategy for long-term maintenance of hypothermia, the technique does offer an inexpensive, practical way to jump-start the cooling process in a manner feasible for critical care transport teams. Further experience is needed to confirm the utility of this approach.

COST OF TRANSPORTATION

The transport of critically ill and injured patients is expensive. Critical care transport services, especially those involved in air medical transport, involve substantial financial investments. Air medical transport operations have significant costs associated with the aircraft, pilots, mechanics, and communications staff, in addition to the medical crew. It is important to understand the broader impact that a critical care transport service may have for an institution.

The decision to operate critical care transport services can be important to the medical center on several levels. Critical care transport services can extend the reach and number of patients that can be served by specialty care available at the receiving institution. This extension of availability is of great clinical benefit to the patients in the service area of a given transport service. Additionally, for the facilities that operate these transport systems, the downstream revenues generated by increased use of its highly specialized resources often offset the costs of the transport and make providing the specialty service cost effective.[21]

Depending on the geographic and demographic makeup of the service area of a tertiary health system, a critical care transport service may be essential to provide a steady supply of patients to the health system.

SUMMARY

Patients who have neurological emergencies often require critical care transport to tertiary care hospitals with the ability to provide specialized neurocritical care, stroke care, or neurosurgical care. Referring physicians should be familiar with the range of possible indications for transporting patients who have neurological emergencies, both to avoid unnecessary transfers and to maximize the potential benefit of transfer for appropriate patients. Referring physicians also must be aware of the capabilities and expertise of the transporting crew. Special characteristics of the critical care transport environment and of the interaction of that environment with victims of neurological emergencies have been reviewed in this article. These interactions are important and should be familiar to all those involved in critical care transport, including the transport teams themselves, and those caring for patients at both referring and receiving hospitals.

REFERENCES

1. Silbergleit R, Burney RE, Nelson K, et al. Long-term air medical services system performance using APACHE-II and mortality benchmarking. Prehosp Emerg Care 2003;7:195–8.
2. Hacke W, Donnan G, Fieschi C, et al. Association of outcome with early stroke treatment: pooled analysis of ATLANTIS, ECASS, and NINDS rt-PA stroke trials. Lancet 2004;363:768–74.
3. Silbergleit R, Scott PA, Lowell MJ, et al. Cost-effectiveness of helicopter transport of stroke patients for thrombolysis. Acad Emerg Med 2003;10:966–72.
4. Alberts MJ, Hademenos G, Latchaw RE, et al. Recommendations for the establishment of primary stroke centers. Brain attack coalition. JAMA 2000;283:3102–9.
5. Stradling D, Yu W, Langdorf ML, et al. Stroke care delivery before vs after JCAHO stroke center certification. Neurology 2007;68:469–70.
6. Silbergleit R, Burney RE, Draper J, et al. Outcome of patients after air medical transport for management of nontraumatic acute intracranial bleeding. Prehosp Disaster Med 1994;9:252–6.
7. Silbergleit R, Dedrick DK, Pape J, et al. Forces acting during air and ground transport on patients stabilized by standard immobilization techniques. Ann Emerg Med 1991;20:875–7.
8. Davis DP, Dunford JV, Poste JC, et al. The impact of hypoxia and hyperventilation on outcome after paramedic rapid sequence intubation of severely head-injured patients. J Trauma 2004;57:1–8 [discussion: 10].
9. Davis DP, Idris AH, Sise MJ, et al. Early ventilation and outcome in patients with moderate to severe traumatic brain injury. Crit Care Med 2006;34:1202–8.
10. Davis DP, Peay J, Serrano JA, et al. The impact of aeromedical response to patients with moderate to severe traumatic brain injury. Ann Emerg Med 2005; 46:115–22.
11. Davis DP, Dunford JV, Ochs M, et al. The use of quantitative end-tidal capnometry to avoid inadvertent severe hyperventilation in patients with head injury after paramedic rapid sequence intubation. J Trauma 2004;56:808–14.

12. Price DD, Wilson SR, Fee ME. Sidestream end-tidal carbon dioxide monitoring during helicopter transport. Air Med J 2007;26:55–9.
13. The Hypothermia after Cardiac Arrest Study Group. Mild therapeutic hypothermia to improve the neurological outcome after cardiac arrest. N Engl J Med 2002;346: 549–56.
14. Bernard SA, Gray TW, Buist MD, et al. Treatment of comatose survivors of out-of-hospital cardiac arrest with induced hypothermia. N Engl J Med 2002; 346:557–63.
15. Majersik JJ, Silbergleit R, Meurer WJ, et al. Public health impact of full implementation of therapeutic hypothermia after cardiac arrest. Resuscitation 2008;77: 189–94.
16. Badjatia N, Bodock M, Guanci M, et al. Rapid infusion of cold saline (4 degrees C) as adjunctive treatment of fever in patients with brain injury. Neurology 2006; 66:1739–41.
17. Bernard S, Buist M, Monteiro O, et al. Induced hypothermia using large volume, ice-cold intravenous fluid in comatose survivors of out-of-hospital cardiac arrest: a preliminary report. Resuscitation 2003;56:9–13.
18. Bernard SA, Rosalion A. Therapeutic hypothermia induced during cardiopulmonary resuscitation using large-volume, ice-cold intravenous fluid. Resuscitation 2008;76:311–3.
19. Kim F, Olsufka M, Longstreth WT Jr, et al. Pilot randomized clinical trial of prehospital induction of mild hypothermia in out-of-hospital cardiac arrest patients with a rapid infusion of 4 degrees C normal saline. Circulation 2007; 115:3064–70.
20. Moore TM, Callaway CW, Hostler D. Core temperature cooling in healthy volunteers after rapid intravenous infusion of cold and room temperature saline solution. Ann Emerg Med 2008;51:153–9.
21. Rosenberg BL, Butz DA, Comstock MC, et al. Aeromedical service: how does it actually contribute to the mission? J Trauma 2003;54:681–8.

Clinical Nihilism in Neuroemergencies

J. Claude Hemphill III, MD, MAS[a,b,c,*], Douglas B. White, MD, MAS[d,e,f,g]

KEYWORDS

- Prognosis • Do-not-resuscitate • Withdrawal of support
- Intracerebral hemorrhage • Traumatic brain injury

Prognostication matters.[1] This is especially true in the context of acute neurologic emergencies. In patients who have acute stroke, severe traumatic brain injury (TBI), or hypoxic-ischemic encephalopathy (HIE) after resuscitation from cardiac arrest, treatment decisions are made not only based on the risk-benefit ratio, but with the consideration of whether any treatment is futile based on poor patient prognosis. Outcome prediction models for these and other acute neurologic conditions have been developed, and some investigators have suggested that these models should be used for early patient triage, including decisions to limit the use of life-sustaining treatments.[2] The initial emergency department evaluation of a patient who has one of these acute neurologic conditions is a critical time point. It is often the point at which physicians (eg, emergency medicine, neurologists, neurosurgeons, intensivists) make that pivotal decision to engage aggressively in evaluation and treatment or whether further treatment seems futile.

Arguments have been made that these early decisions to limit treatment at the time of initial emergency assessment are ethically appropriate (so as to avoid prolonging suffering by delivering medical care that is futile) and financially important (so as to avoid high-cost medical care that has no chance to improve outcome).[3] All these considerations are predicated on the assumption that prognostication is sufficiently

This work was supported by National Institutes of Health (NIH) grants K23NS41240 and U10NS058931 (JCH) and grant KL2RR024130 from the National Center for Research Resources, a component of the NIH and NIH Roadmap for Medical Research (DBW).

[a] Department of Neurology, San Francisco General Hospital, University of California, Room 4M62, 1001 Potrero Avenue, San Francisco, CA 94110, USA
[b] Department of Neurological Surgery, University of California, San Francisco
[c] Neurocritical Care Program, San Francisco General Hospital, University of California
[d] Department of Medicine, University of California, San Francisco
[e] Department of Anesthesia, University of California, San Francisco
[f] UCSF Clinical Ethics Core
[g] University of California, 521 Parnassus Avenue, Suite C-126, Box 0903, San Francisco, CA 94143–0903, USA
* Corresponding author. Department of Neurology, San Francisco General Hospital, Room 4M62, 1001 Potrero Avenue, San Francisco, CA 94110.
E-mail address: chemphill@sfgh.ucsf.edu (J.C. Hemphill).

Emerg Med Clin N Am 27 (2009) 27–37
doi:10.1016/j.emc.2008.08.009
0733-8627/08/$ – see front matter © 2009 Elsevier Inc. All rights reserved.

emed.theclinics.com

accurate and reliable to enable decision making this early after an acute neurologic catastrophe, however. This raises important concerns about how we prognosticate, how we use this information in individual patient decision-making in the emergency setting, and how we communicate this information to patients and their families. Finally, it leads to the fundamental question: Is nihilism an effective treatment strategy in neuroemergencies?

WHAT'S THE PROGNOSIS DOC?

Prognostication is inherent in every new patient encounter regardless of the medical condition being treated or its severity. Patients, and often their families and surrogates, always want to know "how am I going to do?" Although often not explicitly considered as prognostication, when a patient is told that his or her hand laceration is going to heal in several weeks or that his or her headache should be gone by morning, he or she is being offered a prognostic assessment as part of evaluation and treatment. Yet, the importance of prognostication seems more relevant when a patient has a real chance of death or disability. Interestingly, however, the concept of prognostication is often poorly understood and misused in the clinical context.

Prognosis is defined, according to the *Merriam-Webster Dictionary*, as "the prospect of recovery as anticipated from the usual course of disease or peculiarities of the case."[4] Likewise, to prognosticate is "to foretell from signs or symptoms."[5] Prognostication is the act of trying to tell the future. Too often, it is mistakenly taken to be the act of telling what is going to be rather than what may be or is likely to be, however. In clinical practice, prognosis is frequently simplistically considered as a dichotomous outcome: is the prognosis good or bad? Yet, prognostication really involves two different aspects: basically (1) how good do you expect the patient to get, and (2) how sure do you want to be? In the setting of severe TBI, a 90% likelihood of return to work at 6 months may be quite different than a 50% likelihood of living at home under supervision at 1 year. Yet, both represent a prognosis. A prognosis is a probability of a possible outcome. Thus, uncertainty is an inherent aspect of prognostication in all but the most extreme cases. Accepting this uncertainty is central to using prognostic information appropriately in clinical decision making. So, how do we prognosticate in neuroemergencies, and are we good at it?

DOES PROGNOSTIC INFORMATION AFFECT LIFE SUPPORT DECISIONS IN INTENSIVE CARE UNITS?

Murphy and colleagues[6] and Schonwetter and colleagues[7] found that elderly patients substantially overestimated the likelihood of success from cardiopulmonary resuscitation (CPR) and that their willingness to undergo CPR significantly decreased after receiving quantitative data on CPR outcomes. Weeks and colleagues[8] studied patients who had metastatic cancer and found that those who significantly overestimated their chances of 6-month survival were more likely to choose aggressive treatment compared with those with a more accurate understanding, with no improvement in survival. Fried and colleagues[9] found that seriously ill patients' willingness to consent to life support declined substantially as the likelihood of death or severe functional impairment increased. Lloyd and colleagues[10] reported similar findings, with fewer than 25% of patients willing to undergo prolonged life support for a 20% chance of survival; this proportion declined further when the expected functional outcome was poor. Taken together, these studies suggest that misunderstandings about prognosis may lead to use of life support that is inconsistent with patients' preferences. They also suggest that patients do not require prognostic certainty when faced with the decision of whether to continue life support.

Zier and colleagues[11] pursued surrogate decision makers' views of prognostic information. Although all surrogates in the study judged prognostic information to be important, more than half expressed doubt about physicians' prognostic accuracy. Moreover, the study revealed that surrogates use physicians' prognostications as a "cue" to initiate processes that helped them to prepare for a decision to withdraw life support, including emotional preparation, beginning to say goodbye to the patient, and notification of distant family members to come to the hospital. In aggregate, these data suggest that most patients or surrogates in intensive care units (ICUs) neither require absolute prognostic certainty to withdraw life support nor believe that such certainty is possible. In addition, these data suggest that although "brute prognostication" is unlikely to be an effective way to make decisions, physicians' prognostications remain important considerations for surrogates.

OUTCOME PREDICTION IN NEUROEMERGENCIES

Many observational and epidemiologic studies have been published identifying various parameters that are predictive of outcome after acute neuroemergencies. Most of these are composed of clinical, radiologic, and laboratory variables, many of which are available at the time of initial patient evaluation. Various outcomes have been used to develop these models, including short-term mortality and long-term functional outcome. Numerous formal prediction models or algorithms have been developed from these studies for several different conditions, including nontraumatic intracerebral hemorrhage (ICH), severe TBI, and HIE after resuscitation from cardiac arrest.

Nontraumatic ICH remains without a treatment of proved benefit. Predictors of short-term mortality and, to a lesser degree, long-term functional outcome are relatively well described. Most ICH prediction models have found that clinical status, such as that measured by the Glasgow Coma Scale (GCS) score or National Institutes of Health Stroke Scale (NIHSS), and hematoma volume are strong predictors of 30-day mortality risk and longer term functional outcome. Other clinical predictors present in various models include age, presence and volume of intraventricular hemorrhage (IVH), infratentorial hemorrhage location, admission blood pressure, and coagulopathy.[12–16] The most commonly used ICH prediction model, the ICH score, involves a sum score of points assigned for the GCS (3–4 = 2, 5–12 = 1, 13–15 = 0), hematoma volume ($\geq$30 mL = 1, <30 mL = 0), presence of IVH (yes = 1, no = 0), infratentorial origin (yes = 1, no = 0), and patient age $\geq$80 years (yes = 1, no =0).[14] ICH scores may range from 0 to 6, and each increase in the ICH score is associated with an increased risk for 30-day mortality. Although the ICH score was developed to help standardize communication and risk stratification for ICH clinical care and clinical research, the authors have found clinicians increasingly tempted to use this as an early triage tool. Specifically, the first author of this article has had other physicians suggest that patients with an ICH score of 4 (predicted 30-day mortality of 97% in the original cohort) should not receive critical care or interfacility transport because of perceived futility.

There are at least two problems with this approach. First, it assumes that a 3% chance of survival constitutes medical futility. To date, the only widely accepted definitions of futility are those that include only circumstances in which treatment cannot accomplish the intended goals.[17] Second, there is considerable uncertainty around point estimates from such mortality prediction models. The fact that the 95%

confidence interval of the mortality estimate in the previous example extends from 81% to 100% (Hemphill, unpublished data, 2001) emphasizes this point.

In patients who have extensive traumatic injury to the brain, predictors of death or disability include low GCS score after initial resuscitation, findings of intracranial hemorrhage or swelling on CT scan, older age, abnormal pupillary function, and hypotension early after injury.[18] In general, the motor aspect is the most reliable and informative part of the GCS score. Current TBI guidelines emphasize that a low GCS score early after injury lacks precision for precise prediction of a poor outcome, however. Thus, the recognition of uncertainty remains. Interestingly, there have been attempts to develop prediction models that would drive early decisions to limit care in patients who have TBI with a perceived poor prognosis. A mathematic model derived on 672 patients treated at a single center from 1978 to 1993 suggested that long-term prognosis could be sufficiently predicted at 24 hours after TBI accurately enough to terminate life-sustaining treatments in patients unlikely to survive a severe head injury (GCS score $\leq$8).[2] Notably, however, the overall mortality in this cohort at 6 months was 58.8%, which is nearly double that of most other series of patients who have severe TBI.[19–23] Whether the extremely high mortality rate in this modeling study was attributable to physician bias in the care of severely ill patients who had TBI or other factors is unclear. Nevertheless, it does clearly demonstrate the importance of understanding the context in which a particular prediction model is developed and deciding whether it is likely to apply to a specific patient (or population) in which care decisions are being made.

There have been many attempts to predict outcome in comatose survivors of cardiac arrest with HIE. Numerous studies have focused on clinical, neuroimaging, laboratory, and electrophysiologic predictors. A commonly cited study published in 1985 described the outcome of patients with various clinical examination findings at different time points after resuscitation from cardiac arrest.[24] Generally, findings at 3 days after arrest have been considered the most informative. Other studies have examined the likelihood of an unfavorable outcome based on a range of predictors.[25] Importantly, recent practice parameters from the American Academy of Neurology suggested that in the absence of brain death, clinical examination findings at day 3 of absent pupil or corneal reflexes or a motor response that was absent or no better than extensor had a sufficiently low false-positive rate to predict extremely poor long-term functional outcome reliably.[26] This emphasizes that even in the setting of deep coma, some period of waiting is usually desirable to clarify the persistence and validity of clinical examination findings. Whether a trial of aggressive therapy (eg, moderate hypothermia)[27,28] alters these predictive parameters in hypoxic-ischemic coma is not clearly known.

A common finding in these attempts to predict outcome early across various types of neuroemergencies is intuitive. Patients in a coma tend to do worse, especially if they are older. The finding of extensive injury on head imaging studies is also suggestive. The challenge is how to use this information in planning patient treatment. Many of these models and prediction tools described previously have been validated and are used in various forms in the context of current clinical management. Most of the time, however, clinicians prognosticate based not on a specific formal outcome prediction model but, instead, on their own impressions based on experience, knowledge of the medical literature, and clinical intuition. This informal prognostic method is probably really an individual physician's internalized outcome prediction model. A central question is whether this informal method is accurate and consistent, however. Furthermore, recent work has raised the concern that inaccuracy or variability in prognostication could lead to self-fulfilling prophecies of poor outcome.

WHAT IS THE SELF-FULFILLING PROPHECY?

A self-fulfilling prophecy is a prediction that becomes real or true by virtue of having been predicted or expected.[29] The term *self-fulfilling prophecy* is credited to the sociologist Robert K. Merton, who described the self-fulfilling prophecy as "in the beginning, a *false* definition of the situation evoking a new behavior which makes the original false conception come 'true'. This specious validity of the self-fulfilling prophecy perpetuates a reign of error. For the prophet will cite the actual course of events as proof that he was right from the very beginning."[30] This stemmed from a concept described as the Thomas theorem: "If men define situations as real, they are real in their consequences."[31] Even though these are modern terms, the concept of the self-fulfilling prophecy is a familiar and ancient one, as evidenced by its central importance in Shakespeare's *Macbeth* and the Greek legend of Oedipus. Is this relevant to the treatment of neuroemergencies in the twenty-first century? Potentially.

Take an example of a hypothetical cohort of 100 patients with severe stroke in which 70 of them die. Now assume that the death of approximately 70% of these patients was preceded by withdrawal of support.[32] If some proportion (eg, one quarter) of these patients in whom support was withdrawn might actually have survived, the "true" mortality rate of the cohort was not 70% but rather 58%. This would mean that 12 of the 49 patients who underwent withdrawal of support died as a result of a self-fulfilling prophecy. It is probably not possible to determine who among the group those specific 12 patients were, however. Furthermore, any outcome prediction model based on such a cohort would also be based, in part, on the self-fulfilling prophecy that had occurred.

Certainly in neuroemergencies, such as stroke, TBI, and HIE, functional outcome is probably an even more important end point than mortality. However, patients must survive in order to improve. Thus, irrespective of the specific outcome measure chosen in a specific circumstance, the general goal of avoiding a self-fulfilling prophecy of poor outcome remains.

DOES PROGNOSTICATION INFLUENCE OUTCOME?

None of the prediction models developed for neuroemergencies, such as ICH, TBI, or HIE, takes into account factors related to treating physicians, such as their overall patient prognosis or whether they plan to treat aggressively or consider care limitations. Nevertheless, as increasing attention is justifiably being paid to the importance of ethical and compassionate end-of-life care in critical illness,[33] concerns are also being raised about the possibility of self-fulfilling prophecies of death or disability if treatment is limited in patients with a high but not absolute risk for mortality.[34,35]

Why might there be uncertainty? One central tenet is that outcome prediction models (formal or informal) are made from studies of populations of patients but that decisions to limit treatment based on poor prognosis are made on individual patients. Prognosticating outcome in an individual patient using a model developed from a group of patients is inherently uncertain. In fact, prognostic models describe a probability of a specific outcome, such as dead or alive, but an individual patient can only have one of these outcomes. It becomes obvious that if a clinical decision rule is made, such as to withdraw medical support in all patients with greater than 90% risk for death, 100% now die. Prognostication, or at least the application of prognostic data, has changed prognosis.

Empiric evidence suggests this theoretic concern also is a real problem in the care of patients with neurologic emergencies. In a single-center study of 87 patients who had ICH, Becker and colleagues[34] found that the single most important prognostic variable in determining outcome was the level of medical support provided. In fact, withdrawal of support negated the predictive value of all other variables studied. Furthermore, they found wide heterogeneity across different physicians regarding their expectation of prognosis in the same patients. They suggested that treatment limitations, especially withdrawal of life support, might lead to self-fulfilling prophecies of poor outcome.

It is well recognized that heterogeneity exists in the use of various aggressive treatments for ICH, such as surgical hematoma evacuation,[36] and this is not surprising, given the lack of a proven effective treatment and the limited number of large clinical trials that have been performed in ICH.[37–39] This raises the question as to whether there is also heterogeneity in the use of measures to limit care early after ICH and whether this influences outcome. The 1983 US President's Commission on Deciding to Forgo Life-Sustaining Treatment emphasized that a do-not-resuscitate (DNR) policy should ensure that the DNR order has no implications for any other treatment decisions.[40] In practice, however, DNR orders are often the first step in a continuum of care limitation.[41] Additionally, variability has been found in the use of DNR orders.[42,43]

Hemphill and colleagues[44] hypothesized that the rate at which a hospital uses DNR orders within the first 24 hours of admission for ICH influences patient outcome irrespective of other hospital and patient characteristics. From a California-wide hospital discharge database, 8233 patients who had ICH and were treated at 234 different hospitals were identified. Early DNR orders were one of the most common interventions, with 25% of patients having DNR orders within 24 hours of hospital admission. This was much higher than the proportion of patients who underwent aggressive interventions, such as surgical hematoma evacuation or ventriculostomy placement. Of note, the rate at which a hospital used DNR orders within 24 hours of patient admission for ICH increased the odds of individual patient death, even after adjusting for patient characteristics, such as age, use of mechanical ventilation (a surrogate for coma), and hospital characteristics (eg, number of patients who had ICH treated, designation as a teaching hospital or trauma center). Even more importantly, there was an interaction between an individual patient's DNR status and the hospital DNR rate. This means that not only does the individual patient's DNR status matter but that it matters which hospital the patient who has DNR orders is admitted to. Different hospitals (and presumably physicians) used DNR orders differently, and this influenced a patient's risk for dying. These findings of early care limitations influencing outcome in acute ICH have been confirmed by others in a separate cohort of patients in Texas.[45]

This type of analysis suggests several things. First, use of measures to limit treatment early is extremely common, at least in ICH. Second, it is not the DNR orders themselves that are leading to patient death. In fact, DNR orders should have no effect on patient outcome unless the patient has cardiac arrest. Rather, high use of early DNR orders at a hospital is a marker of an overall nonaggressive approach to ICH patients in general, and this suggests that there is something about the milieu of care in a hospital that influences outcome, potentially in a very negative way. Third, it clearly demonstrates that nihilism is an ineffective treatment strategy.

Likewise, for TBI, the ability to prognosticate accurately and precisely early has been questioned. Kaufmann and colleagues[46] performed a study in which 100 consecutive patients who had severe TBI were evaluated to determine whether the expected prognosis on day 1 was accurate. Interestingly, it was found that an experienced neurosurgeon underestimated favorable 1-year outcomes and overestimated poor outcomes. Notably, an experienced neuroradiologist did the opposite, overestimating favorable outcomes and underestimating poor outcomes. These investigators concluded that in severe head injury, it was not possible to predict outcome reliably on the first day with sufficient accuracy to guide management, at least for purposes of unilaterally limiting treatment.

It is noteworthy that these issues are not limited to acute neurologic emergencies but apply to general critical care as well. Rocker and colleagues[47] found that physician estimates of a patient having a less than 10% likelihood of surviving to ICU discharge were associated with subsequent life support limitation. Furthermore, these estimates were more predictive of ICU mortality than illness severity itself. In a different study, Frick and colleagues[48] found that physicians tended to be overly pessimistic about survival and quality of life of ICU patients. Additionally, ICU nurses tended to suggest treatment withdrawal more often than physicians for patients who ultimately survived.

These emerging studies of the association of early treatment limitation and outcome coupled with increasing recognition of the challenges of precisely prognosticating outcome early in neuroemergencies have engendered concern regarding how to balance issues of ensuring aggressive care for those patients who might benefit while avoiding the costs (financially and psychologically) of futile care. Many approaches now advocate a trial of "aggressive treatment" for at least some period in these neuroemergencies, such as ICH, TBI, and HIE, if this is congruent with the patient's wishes. The 2007 revision of the American Stroke Association Guidelines for the Management of Spontaneous Intracerebral Hemorrhage in Adults includes a new recommendation to carefully consider aggressive full care during the first 24 hours after ICH onset and to postpone new DNR orders during that time.[49] Perhaps most importantly, these emerging concerns have placed renewed focus on the goals of prognostication, and how this interacts with surrogate decision making in the setting of acute neurologic catastrophes.

WHAT ARE WE TRYING TO ACHIEVE WITH PROGNOSTICATION?

A central tenet of American bioethics is that medical care should reflect the values of the patient.[50] Although it is true that surrogates struggle to enact this standard of decision making for incapacitated patients because of their difficulty in knowing what the patient would choose for himself or herself, the problem is only compounded by misunderstandings about prognosis. Surrogates who are inaccurately pessimistic about prognosis may opt to forego treatment that the patient may have desired. Surrogates who have an overly optimistic view may choose life support in a setting in which the patient would not want it. In both circumstances, patient-centered care is compromised. Moreover, when life support is continued in patients who would not choose it, this may create problems at a societal level, because critical care services in the United States are an expensive and limited resource, for which demand sometimes exceeds supply.[51] The problem of resource scarcity is likely to grow as the aging population increases.[52]

The most important role for prognostication in acute neuroemergencies is in communicating risk. Prognostication is intrinsically linked to the process of communication in the care of severely ill patients. It is important to contrast this emphasis on communication and shared decision making with some of the potentially darker aspects of prognostication, especially those that might reinforce early nihilism. The use of prognostic information to limit initial and early care because of physician nihilism attributable to anticipated futility is potentially problematic if this is not congruent with the patient's (or family's) wishes to attempt aggressive care, especially if the true prognosis is perhaps less certain than that assumed by the physician. Because physicians generally cannot be compelled to provide specific medical or surgical interventions that are futile, the accuracy of prognosis is central to conflicts that arise between patient (or family) wishes and physicians about the intensity of care to be attempted. An additional argument frequently made is that high health care costs might be limited by limiting intensive care at the end of life. Although this might seem intuitively correct when considering an individual patient's health care costs, this may not be the case. Luce and Rubenfeld[53] suggested that the fixed costs of ICU beds; hospital wards; and personnel, such as nursing and respiratory therapists, outweigh the variable costs of an individual patient's hospitalization and that the only way to reduce costs truly in this manner may be to close beds and fire personnel.

The authors strongly favor using prognostic information to support shared decision making with patients and families early in the setting of an acute neuroemergency rather than as a way to usurp their autonomy and deny or force care. This usually includes explaining, and even embracing, the uncertainty inherent in prognostication. Thus, the focus is increasingly on principles of communication and setting the stage for decision making to come.

Many issues remain to be clarified. If prognostication at the time of an acute neuroemergency is too imprecise to help inform medical decisions, at what point is it sufficiently accurate? Is the concept of prognosis as a range of possible outcomes with various probabilities too complex for nonmedical patients and families to understand? If we try a trial of aggressive treatment, do we "miss" a window in which to withdraw support in a severely injured patient? These are all concerns that have been communicated to the authors by staff in their own medical centers. Yet, these concerns really bring one back to the importance of communication with patients and families in the context of acute illness, especially high-risk acute catastrophes, such as stroke, TBI, and cardiac arrest. The challenge is how to implement this in a medically and ethically sound way.

SUMMARY

The acute management of patients who have neuroemergencies, such as stroke, TBI, and HIE after cardiac arrest, is not a simple task. Only a small number of interventions have been clearly shown in randomized trials to be of benefit, yet decisions regarding optimal care have to be made in every patient, and often for numerous issues. Many times the first decision faced by physicians in this context is whether to "engage" by pursuing a trial of aggressive treatment or to "retreat" and initiate approaches to limit treatment based on perceived poor prognosis. A better appreciation of the imprecision of early prognostication and the potential deleterious effects of early treatment limitations has served to emphasize the challenge of decision making at this early critical point. Yet, even in the absence of a treatment of proven benefit, nihilism is not an effective overall treatment strategy.

REFERENCES

1. Johnston SC. Prognostication matters. Muscle Nerve 2000;23(6):839–42.
2. Mamelak AN, Pitts LH, Damron S. Predicting survival from head trauma 24 hours after injury: a practical method with therapeutic implications. J Trauma 1996; 41(1):91–9.
3. Fries JF, Koop CE, Beadle CE, et al. Reducing health care costs by reducing the need and demand for medical services. The Health Project Consortium. N Engl J Med 1993;329(5):321–5.
4. Available at: http://www.merriam-webster.com/dictionary/prognosis. Accessed July 16, 2008.

5. Available at: http://www.merriam-webster.com/dictionary/prognosticate. Accessed July 16, 2008.
6. Murphy DJ, Burrows D, Santilli S, et al. The influence of the probability of survival on patients' preferences regarding cardiopulmonary resuscitation. N Engl J Med 1994;330(8):545–9.
7. Schonwetter RS, Walker RM, Kramer DR, et al. Resuscitation decision making in the elderly: the value of outcome data. J Gen Intern Med 1993;8(6):295–300.
8. Weeks JC, Cook EF, O'Day SJ, et al. Relationship between cancer patients' predictions of prognosis and their treatment preferences. JAMA 1998;279(21): 1709–14.
9. Fried TR, Bradley EH, Towle VR, et al. Understanding the treatment preferences of seriously ill patients. N Engl J Med 2002;346(14):1061–6.
10. Lloyd CB, Nietert PJ, Silvestri GA. Intensive care decision making in the seriously ill and elderly. Crit Care Med 2004;32(3):649–54.
11. Zier LS, Burack JH, Micco G, et al. Doubt and belief in physicians' ability to prognosticate during critical illness: the perspective of surrogate decision makers. Crit Care Med 2008;36(8):2341–7.
12. Broderick JP, Brott TG, Duldner JE, et al. Volume of intracerebral hemorrhage. A powerful and easy-to-use predictor of 30-day mortality. Stroke 1993;24(7): 987–93.
13. Flibotte JJ, Hagan N, O'Donnell J, et al. Warfarin, hematoma expansion, and outcome of intracerebral hemorrhage. Neurology 2004;63(6):1059–64.
14. Hemphill JC 3rd, Bonovich DC, Besmertis L, et al. The ICH score: a simple, reliable grading scale for intracerebral hemorrhage. Stroke 2001;32(4):891–7.
15. Lisk DR, Pasteur W, Rhoades H, et al. Early presentation of hemispheric intracerebral hemorrhage: prediction of outcome and guidelines for treatment allocation. Neurology 1994;44(1):133–9.
16. Tuhrim S, Horowitz DR, Sacher M, et al. Validation and comparison of models predicting survival following intracerebral hemorrhage. Crit Care Med 1995;23(5): 950–4.
17. Consensus statement of the Society of Critical Care Medicine's Ethics Committee regarding futile and other possibly inadvisable treatments. Crit Care Med 1997; 25(5):887–91.
18. Management and prognosis of severe traumatic brain injury. Brain Trauma Foundation; 2000.
19. Fearnside MR, Cook RJ, McDougall P, et al. The Westmead Head Injury Project. Physical and social outcomes following severe head injury. Br J Neurosurg 1993; 7(6):643–50.
20. Fearnside MR, Cook RJ, McDougall P, et al. The Westmead Head Injury Project outcome in severe head injury. A comparative analysis of pre-hospital, clinical and CT variables. Br J Neurosurg 1993;7(3):267–79.
21. Marshall LF, Becker DP, Bowers SA, et al. The National Traumatic Coma Data Bank. Part 1: design, purpose, goals, and results. J Neurosurg 1983;59(2): 276–84.
22. Murray GD, Teasdale GM, Braakman R, et al. The European Brain Injury Consortium survey of head injuries. Acta Neurochir (Wien) 1999;141(3):223–36.
23. Myburgh JA, Cooper DJ, Finfer SR, et al. Epidemiology and 12-month outcomes from traumatic brain injury in Australia and New Zealand. J Trauma 2008;64(4): 854–62.
24. Levy DE, Caronna JJ, Singer BH, et al. Predicting outcome from hypoxic-ischemic coma. JAMA 1985;253(10):1420–6.

25. Booth CM, Boone RH, Tomlinson G, et al. Is this patient dead, vegetative, or severely neurologically impaired? Assessing outcome for comatose survivors of cardiac arrest. JAMA 2004;291(7):870–9.
26. Wijdicks EF, Hijdra A, Young GB, et al. Practice parameter: prediction of outcome in comatose survivors after cardiopulmonary resuscitation (an evidence-based review): report of the Quality Standards Subcommittee of the American Academy of Neurology. Neurology 2006;67(2):203–10.
27. The Hypothermia After Cardiac Arrest Study Group. Mild therapeutic hypothermia to improve the neurologic outcome after cardiac arrest. N Engl J Med 2002;346(8):549–56.
28. Bernard SA, Gray TW, Buist MD, et al. Treatment of comatose survivors of out-of-hospital cardiac arrest with induced hypothermia. N Engl J Med 2002;346(8):557–63.
29. Available at: http://www.merriam-webster.com/dictionary/self-fulfilling. Accessed August 5, 2008.
30. Merton RK. Social theory and social structure. New York: Free Press; 1968. p. 477.
31. Thomas WI. The child in America: behavior problems and programs. New York: Alfred A. Knopf; 1928. p. 572.
32. Zurasky JA, Aiyagari V, Zazulia AR, et al. Early mortality following spontaneous intracerebral hemorrhage. Neurology 2005;64(4):725–7.
33. Levy MM, McBride DL. End-of-life care in the intensive care unit: state of the art in 2006. Crit Care Med 2006;34(11 Suppl):S306–8.
34. Becker KJ, Baxter AB, Cohen WA, et al. Withdrawal of support in intracerebral hemorrhage may lead to self-fulfilling prophecies. Neurology 2001;56(6):766–72.
35. Hemphill JC 3rd. Do-not-resuscitate orders, unintended consequences, and the ripple effect. Crit Care 2007;11(2):121.
36. Gregson BA, Mendelow AD. International variations in surgical practice for spontaneous intracerebral hemorrhage. Stroke 2003;34(11):2593–7.
37. Lyden PD, Shuaib A, Lees KR, et al. Safety and tolerability of NXY-059 for acute intracerebral hemorrhage: the CHANT Trial. Stroke 2007;38(8):2262–9.
38. Mayer SA, Brun NC, Begtrup K, et al. Efficacy and safety of recombinant activated factor VII for acute intracerebral hemorrhage. N Engl J Med 2008; 358(20):2127–37.
39. Mendelow AD, Gregson BA, Fernandes HM, et al. Early surgery versus initial conservative treatment in patients with spontaneous supratentorial intracerebral haematomas in the International Surgical Trial in Intracerebral Haemorrhage (STICH): a randomised trial. Lancet 2005;365(9457):387–97.
40. President's Commission for the Study of Ethical Problems in Medicine and Biomedical and Behavioral Research. Deciding to forego life-sustaining treatment. U.S. Government Printing Office; 1983.
41. Vetsch G, Uehlinger DE, Zuercher-Zenklusen RM. DNR orders at a tertiary care hospital—are they appropriate? Swiss Med Wkly 2002;132(15–16):190–6.
42. Shepardson LB, Gordon HS, Ibrahim SA, et al. Racial variation in the use of do-not-resuscitate orders. J Gen Intern Med 1999;14(1):15–20.
43. Shepardson LB, Youngner SJ, Speroff T, et al. Variation in the use of do-not-resuscitate orders in patients with stroke. Arch Intern Med 1997;157(16):1841–7.
44. Hemphill JC 3rd, Newman J, Zhao S, et al. Hospital usage of early do-not-resuscitate orders and outcome after intracerebral hemorrhage. Stroke 2004;35(5):1130–4.

45. Zahuranec DB, Brown DL, Lisabeth LD, et al. Early care limitations independently predict mortality after intracerebral hemorrhage. Neurology 2007;68(20):1651–7.
46. Kaufmann MA, Buchmann B, Scheidegger D, et al. Severe head injury: should expected outcome influence resuscitation and first-day decisions? Resuscitation 1992;23(3):199–206.
47. Rocker G, Cook D, Sjokvist P, et al. Clinician predictions of intensive care unit mortality. Crit Care Med 2004;32(5):1149–54.
48. Frick S, Uehlinger DE, Zuercher Zenklusen RM. Medical futility: predicting outcome of intensive care unit patients by nurses and doctors—a prospective comparative study. Crit Care Med 2003;31(2):456–61.
49. Broderick J, Connolly S, Feldmann E, et al. Guidelines for the management of spontaneous intracerebral hemorrhage in adults: 2007 update: a guideline from the American Heart Association/American Stroke Association Stroke Council, High Blood Pressure Research Council, and the Quality of Care and Outcomes in Research Interdisciplinary Working Group. Stroke 2007;38(6):2001–23.
50. Truog RD, Campbell ML, Curtis JR, et al. Recommendations for end-of-life care in the intensive care unit: a consensus statement by the American College [corrected] of Critical Care Medicine. Crit Care Med 2008;36(3):953–63.
51. Teres D. Civilian triage in the intensive care unit: the ritual of the last bed. Crit Care Med 1993;21(4):598–606.
52. Danis M. Improving end-of-life care in the intensive care unit: what's to be learned from outcomes research? New Horiz 1998;6(1):110–8.
53. Luce JM, Rubenfeld GD. Can health care costs be reduced by limiting intensive care at the end of life? Am J Respir Crit Care Med 2002;165(6):750–4.

Vertigo and Dizziness in the Emergency Department

Kevin A. Kerber, MD

KEYWORDS

- Vertigo • Dizziness • Emergency department • Stroke
- Vestibular neuritis • Benign paroxysmal positional vertigo

Dizziness can be a problematic presentation in the emergency department, both from a diagnostic and a management standpoint. Dizziness is among the most common reasons that patients present for an evaluation.[1] In terms of signs and symptoms, overlap exists among the many potential causes. The report of symptoms can be vague, inconsistent, or unreliable.[2] Life-threatening disorders can masquerade as benign disorders,[3–7] but tests ordered to screen for life-threatening disorders are often insensitive.[8]

Patients presenting with vertigo and dizziness in the emergency department typically fall into one of the following three categories: acute severe dizziness, recurrent attacks of dizziness, or recurrent positional dizziness (**Table 1**). A benign peripheral vestibular disorder is the most common cause within each of these categories and fortunately each of these disorders—vestibular neuritis, benign paroxysmal positional vertigo, and Meniere's disease—is characterized by unique features allowing for a bedside diagnosis. Often, the most effective way to "rule-out" a life-threatening disorder is to "rule-in" one of these peripheral vestibular disorders. Because of this, it is critical that physicians can identify the key features of these three common peripheral vestibular disorders. The time to consider a sinister disorder as the cause is when the presentation is atypical for a peripheral vestibular disorder or when other red flags are identified (**Fig. 1**).

This article focuses on the categories of vertigo and dizziness presentations and the peripheral vestibular disorder that corresponds to each category.

ACUTE SEVERE DIZZINESS

The patient who presents with sudden onset severe dizziness, in the absence of prior similar episodes, has the "acute severe dizziness" presentation. Patients with acute

Dr. Kerber is supported by Grant No. K23 RR02409 from the National Institutes of Health, National Center for Research Resources.
Department of Neurology, University of Michigan Health System, 1500 East Medical Center Drive, TC 1920/0316, Ann Arbor, MI 48109-0316, USA
E-mail address: kakerber@med.umich.edu

Emerg Med Clin N Am 27 (2009) 39–50
doi:10.1016/j.emc.2008.09.002
0733-8627/08/$ – see front matter © 2009 Elsevier Inc. All rights reserved.

Table 1
Summary of the features of the most common categories of dizziness presentations

Dizziness Presentation Category	Main Symptoms	Peripheral Vestibular Signs	Central Nervous System Signs[b]	Potential Causes
Acute severe dizziness	Sudden onset, severe and constant dizziness, nausea and vomiting, and imbalance	Unidirectional spontaneous nystagmus, positive head-thrust test	Down-beat or bidirectional gaze-evoked nystagmus, severe imbalance	PV: Vestibular neuritis CNS: Stroke
Recurrent positional dizziness	Dizziness attacks triggered by head movements	-Attacks last less than 1 minute. Normal between attacks. -Dix-Hallpike test: Burst of upbeat torsional nystagmus. -Epley maneuver: Resolution of signs and symptoms[a]	-Attacks can be of short or long duration. Less severe dizziness symptoms may persist between attacks. -Dix-Hallpike test: Persistent down-beating nystagmus or pure torsional nystagmus. -Epley maneuver: No effect.	PV: BPPV CNS: Chiari malformation, cerebellar tumor, degenerative ataxia.
Recurrent attacks of dizziness	Spontaneous attacks of dizziness	Duration: >20 minutes to hours. Associated unilateral hearing loss, roaring tinnitus, or ear fullness	Duration: Minutes. New onset and crescendo pattern	PV: Meniere's disease CNS: TIA

Abbreviations: BPPV, benign paroxysmal positional vertigo; CNS = central nervous system; PV = peripheral vestibular; TIA = transient ischemic attack.
[a] See text for details regarding less common types of BPPV.
[b] Any other CNS symptom as well (speech alteration, focal weakness, focal sensory features).

severe dizziness appear ill because of the dizziness and accompanying nausea and vomiting. Impaired ability to walk is also common. Although rigorous epidemiologic studies are lacking, the most common cause is an acute lesion, presumed viral in origin, of the vestibular nerve on one side, so-called vestibular neuritis.[9] The mechanism underlying vestibular neuritis is similar to that of Bell's palsy. The seventh cranial nerve is affected in Bell's palsy, whereas the eighth cranial nerve is affected in vestibular

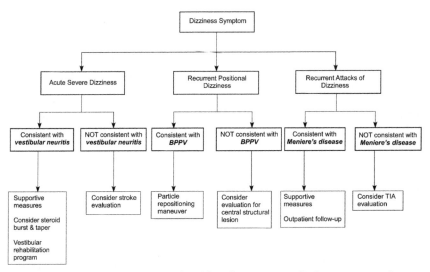

Fig. 1. Diagnostic and management algorithm for common dizziness presentation categories. BPPV, benign paroxysmal positional vertigo; TIA, transient ischemic attack.

neuritis. Patients with vestibular neuritis nearly always report true vertigo, which is characteristically described as visualized spinning of the environment. The symptoms are typically severe for 1 to 2 days with gradual resolution over weeks to months. It is exceedingly rare to have more than one bout of vestibular neuritis, so an alternative diagnosis should be considered whenever more than one episode is reported.

It is now clear that a small stroke within the posterior fossa can present as acute severe dizziness, closely mimicking vestibular neuritis.[3–5] The first step to distinguishing vestibular neuritis from stroke is asking the patient about other neurologic symptoms such as focal numbness, focal weakness, or slurred speech. Mild double vision can result from a peripheral vestibular lesion so this symptom is not a reliable discriminator. The next step is the physical examination. Patients with vestibular neuritis have highly characteristic examination features. Only in an extremely rare case can all of the vestibular neuritis examination features be mimicked by a stroke.

Nystagmus in Acute Severe Dizziness Presentations

Nystagmus is a term used to describe alternating slow and fast movements of the eyes. These alternating movements give the appearance that the eyes are beating toward one or more directions. Patients with vestibular neuritis have a peripheral vestibular pattern of nystagmus. In this setting, the peripheral vestibular pattern is a unidirectional, principally horizontal pattern of nystagmus. This description means that the nystagmus beats in only one direction (ie, a left-beating nystagmus never converts to right-beating, or a right-beating nystagmus never converts to left-beating). Conversely, bidirectional gaze-evoked nystagmus (ie, right beating nystagmus present with gaze toward the right, and left-beating nystagmus present with gaze toward the left side) is a central nervous system pattern of nystagmus.[10] Other central nervous system patterns are pure torsional nystagmus or spontaneous vertical (typically downbeat) nystagmus. With an acute peripheral vestibular lesion, the only pattern of nystagmus that can result is unidirectional nystagmus. In acute severe dizziness presentations, any other pattern should be considered a central nervous system sign. Patients often prefer to keep their eyes closed early on, but the eyes should be opened and the pattern of nystagmus defined.

Nystagmus in vestibular neuritis is spontaneous (ie, present in primary gaze) for at least the first several hours of symptoms. Following this initial time period, the nystagmus may be identified only during gaze testing (ie, having the patient look to each side) or if visual fixation is blocked. Patients can suppress peripheral vestibular nystagmus by visual fixation on a target, so removing the patient's ability to fixate can bring out the spontaneous nystagmus. The simplest way to block fixation is to place a blank sheet of paper a few inches in front of the patient and then observe for spontaneous nystagmus from the side.

The reason for the characteristic pattern of nystagmus in vestibular neuritis is an imbalance in the peripheral vestibular signals to the brain. Normally, the peripheral vestibular system on each side has a baseline firing rate of action potentials that functions to drive the eyes toward the other side. When the peripheral vestibular system on each side is intact, the input from each side is balance so the eyes remain stationary. When an acute lesion occurs on one side, the input from the opposite side is unopposed. As a result, the eyes will be "pushed" toward the lesioned side. This movement of the eyes is the slow phase of nystagmus. When the eyes reach a critical point off center, the brain responds by generating a corrective eye movement to move the eyes back. This is the fast phase of nystagmus. Because the direction of the fast phase gives the appearance that the eyes are beating in that direction, an acute left peripheral vestibular lesion leads to spontaneous right-beating nystagmus. Over time, the asymmetry resolves or the brain compensates for the asymmetry.

The Head-Thrust Test

A recently described bedside test, the "head-thrust test," is now an important component of the bedside evaluation in acute severe dizziness presentations.[11,12] The test allows the examiner to assess the vestibulo-ocular reflex (VOR) on each side. The VOR is the component of the vestibular system that triggers eye movements in response to stimulation. In different settings, the VOR has long been tested using the doll's eye test of the coma examination and caloric stimulation (ie, the laboratory caloric test or the bedside cold caloric test in a comatose patient). To test the VOR using the head thrust test, the examiner stands in front of the patient and grasps the patient's head with both hands. The patient is instructed to focus on the examiner's nose and then the examiner initiates a quick 5- to 10-degree movement of the patient's head to one side. When there is a lesion of the VOR on one side, as occurs with vestibular neuritis, a corrective eye movement (ie, a corrective "saccade") back to the examiner's nose is seen after the head is moved toward the affected side.[12] In contrast and serving as an internal control, the eyes will stay on target (ie, the examiner's nose) after the head thrust test toward the normal side because the VOR is intact on that side. These features can be appreciated even when spontaneous nystagmus is present. The reason for the corrective saccade with a peripheral vestibular lesion is rooted in the physiology of the vestibular system.[10] When the head is moved quickly in one direction, the reflex (ie, the VOR) that moves the eyes toward the opposite direction is generated by the side the head moved toward. Thus a patient with vestibular neuritis of the left side will present with right-beating unidirectional nystagmus and have a positive head thrust test with movements toward the left side.

Vascular Causes of Acute Severe Dizziness

Although vestibular neuritis is the most common cause of the acute dizziness presentation, no laboratory or imaging test exists to confirm a viral etiology. A peripheral vestibular lesion can be caused by a vascular occlusion of the blood supply to the peripheral vestibular components, although presumably this cause is much less common.

Stroke should be a serious consideration in the patient who presents with the acute dizziness presentation. Dizziness is a symptom of stroke in 50% of stroke presentations.[13] Most stroke patients that report dizziness as a symptom have other prominent central nervous system features, but a small stroke of the cerebellum or brain stem can present with isolated dizziness (ie, dizziness without other accompanying central nervous system signs or symptoms). In a population-based study, about 3% of patients with dizziness had a stroke etiology, but less than 1% of patients with isolated dizziness had stroke as the etiology.[14] However, a prospective study of 24 patients with acute severe dizziness reported six patients (25%) with stroke etiology.[3] Patients with stroke presenting as isolated dizziness may report imbalance, true vertigo, a more vague dizziness sensation, or a combination of these. Nausea and vomiting are also common, as they are with vestibular neuritis. Unfortunately, computerized tomography (CT) scans are an extremely insensitive test for acute stroke presentations in general,[15] and particularly so for infarction within the posterior fossa.[16,17] A stroke within the posterior fossa may not appear on a CT scan for days or weeks because of artifacts or poor resolution. Because of this, CT should never be considered as a means of excluding stroke. Magnetic resonance imaging (MRI) is a much more sensitive test, but is not a practical test to screen for stroke in emergency department dizziness presentations. Like CT, the sensitivity of the test is the lowest for stroke of the posterior fossa.[18]

The key features discriminating stroke from vestibular neuritis are the pattern of nystagmus and the results of the head thrust test. Down-beating nystagmus or bidirectional gaze-evoked nystagmus are both immediate indications that the localization must be in the central nervous system. These patterns are not caused by lesions of the peripheral vestibular system. This is the reason that an examination of ocular movements is required before a diagnosis is even considered. Another highly suspicious pattern of nystagmus is a pure torsional pattern. There are now case reports of patients who have unidirectional horizontal nystagmus and a stroke etiology so the pattern of nystagmus should not be the sole criterion.[3–5] A patient with unidirectional nystagmus, a positive head thrust in the direction opposite the fast phase of nystagmus, and no other neurologic features can be diagnosed with vestibular neuritis with a high level of certainty. It would take a well-placed and small stroke to cause the peripheral vestibular pattern of nystagmus and a corresponding positive head thrust test without any other central nervous system features. Although all patients with vestibular neuritis are unsteady walking, the inability to walk is another red flag.[5] Finally, a person's risk for stroke based on stroke risk factors should be considered. Although no validated scale exists to grade stroke risk based on stroke risk factors in this population, a stroke workup is reasonable in patients with a high risk for stroke. One should not be overreliant on stroke risk factors as discriminators, however, since other stroke mechanisms, such as arterial dissection, occur in the absence of stroke risk factors.

Management of Acute Severe Dizziness

The management of the acute dizziness presentation begins with supportive care. If stroke is suspected then a neuroimaging study should be considered. Although CT could serve as the initial study, a normal result on CT should provide little confidence that stroke can be excluded. In this situation, an MRI or hospital admission for close observation should be considered. If stroke is confirmed to be the cause and the patient presents within 3 hours of onset, thrombolytic treatment should be considered. A short course of corticosteroids should be considered for patients with vestibular neuritis. A randomized controlled trial showed that patients with vestibular neuritis treated with corticosteroids within 3 days of symptom onset had a higher likelihood of recovery of the peripheral vestibular caloric response at 12 months.[19] However, this study did not test whether the patient's functional or symptomatic outcome improved, and corticosteroids are not without potential side effects. After the initial severe symptomatic time period, it is important that patients resume activities because this helps the brain to compensate for the asymmetry of vestibular signals. A formal vestibular therapy program has been shown in a randomized trial to improve outcomes in patients with vestibular neuritis.[20]

RECURRENT POSITIONAL DIZZINESS

Patients with positional dizziness have symptoms triggered by certain head positions. In acute presentations, patients are often more frightened by symptoms than debilitated by them.

Benign paroxysmal positional vertigo (BPPV) is the likely cause in patients reporting brief recurrent attacks of dizziness triggered by changes in head position. It is important to recognize this cause because it can be readily treated at the bedside and because identification of the key features is the most effective way to exclude a central nervous system cause of positional dizziness. Important points about BPPV are that the dizziness episodes last less than 1 minute and patients are normal in between episodes. Sometimes nausea or a mild lightheadedness can persist longer than 1 minute, but any patient reporting positional dizziness lasting longer than 1 minute should be carefully scrutinized for other potential causes. A patient with dizziness from any cause will feel worse with certain position changes, but the patient with BPPV has dizziness that is triggered by positional changes and then returns to normal between attacks. Patients with vestibular neuritis are often misclassified as BPPV because the symptoms improve when the patient remains still and worsen with movement, but that is very different from the patient who returns to normal at rest.

BPPV occurs when calcium carbonate debris dislodge from the otoconial membrane in the inner ear and then inadvertently enter a semicircular canal.[21] The debris is typically free-floating in the canal so that head movements will trigger the symptom. The most common semicircular canal affected is the posterior canal because of its anatomic location. However, the particles can also enter the horizontal canal, or very rarely the anterior canal. It is important to be aware of the different variants of BPPV since each has unique examination features.[22] The most common triggers for BPPV episodes are extending the head back to look up (top shelf vertigo), turning over in bed, or getting in and out of bed. Posterior canal BPPV is the most important type to be able to identify because it is the most common type.

Positional Testing and Particle Repositioning

When the patient with posterior canal BPPV is placed in the head-hanging position (Dix-Hallpike test) with the head turned toward the affected side, a burst of upbeat and torsional nystagmus is seen (**Fig. 2**). Turning the head toward one side for the Dix-Hallpike test lines the plane of the posterior canal on that side up with the movement of the test. The duration of nystagmus is typically 15 to 25 seconds. The Epley maneuver, a curative bedside maneuver, can then be used to reposition the debris.[21,23] Success of the maneuver can be confirmed by re-testing. If nystagmus continues to be triggered by the Dix Hallpike test, the Epley maneuver can be repeated.

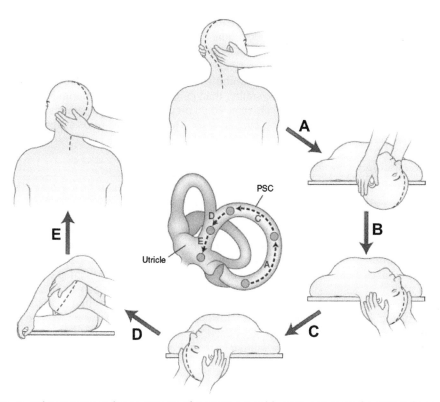

Fig. 2. Epley maneuver for treatment of posterior canal benign paroxysmal positional vertigo affecting the right ear. The procedure can be reversed for treating the left ear. The labyrinth in the center shows the position of the debris as it moves around the posterior semicircular canal (PSC) and into the utricle (UT). The patient is seated upright, with head facing the examiner, who is standing on the right. (A) The patient is then rapidly moved to head-hanging right position (Dix-Hallpike test). This position is maintained until the nystagmus ceases. (B) The examiner moves to the head of the table, repositioning hands as shown. (C) The head is rotated quickly to the left with right ear upward. This position is maintained for 30 seconds. (D) The patient rolls onto the left side while the examiner rapidly rotates the head leftward until the nose is directed toward the floor. This position is then held for 30 seconds. (E) The patient is rapidly lifted into the sitting position, now facing left. The entire sequence should be repeated until no nystagmus can be elicited. Following the maneuver, the patient is instructed to avoid head-hanging positions to prevent the debris from reentering the posterior canal. (*From* Rakel RE. Conn's current therapy 1995. Philadelphia: WB Saunders; 1995. p. 839; with permission.)

When the particles are in the horizontal canal, the nystagmus triggered by head movement is a horizontal nystagmus rather than the vertical-torsional nystagmus seen with BPPV of the posterior canal.[22] If the patient lies supine and turns the head to either side, thus in the plane of the horizontal canal, nystagmus will be triggered. The two potential patterns of nystagmus in horizontal canal BPPV are (1) right-beating nystagmus after head turns toward the right side, then left-beating nystagmus after head turns toward the left side, and (2) left-beating nystagmus after head turns toward the right side and right-beating nystagmus after head turns toward the left side. Which pattern occurs depends on where the debris is located within the horizontal canal. The nystagmus of horizontal canal BPPV typically lasts longer than nystagmus triggered by posterior canal BPPV.[22] BPPV from the horizontal canal can be more difficult to treat than posterior canal BPPV. A common repositioning strategy is to have the patient roll toward the unaffected side (360 degrees) in 90-degree increments.[24] The unaffected side is generally the side that triggers less severe nystagmus. Another approach is simply to instruct the patient to lie on the unaffected side for hours, which can be done at home rather than in the emergency department.[25]

BPPV of the anterior canal is quite rare. When present the Dix-Hallpike test will trigger a short burst of down-beating nystagmus.[22] This cause will also respond to the Epley maneuver.

Central Positional Dizziness

Central positional vertigo stems from a lesion of the cerebellum or the brainstem. Positional vertigo and nystagmus are common features of a Chiari malformation, cerebellar tumor, multiple sclerosis, migraine vertigo, and degenerative ataxia disorders. As with the acute dizziness presentations, the key to distinguishing a central nervous system disorder from a peripheral vestibular disorder is the pattern of nystagmus. The most common pattern of central positional nystagmus is pure down-beating nystagmus that lasts as long as the position is held. Pure torsional nystagmus is another type of central positional nystagmus. The pattern of nystagmus seen with horizontal canal BPPV can also be caused by a central lesion. A general rule is that a central nervous system cause of positional nystagmus should be considered whenever the pattern of nystagmus is a persistent down-beating nystagmus, pure-torsional nystagmus, or whenever the nystagmus is refractory to repositioning maneuvers.

RECURRENT ATTACKS OF DIZZINESS

Patients with recurrent attacks of dizziness will report prior episodes that were similar to the current attack. The duration of the attacks is highly variable but can be helpful in discriminating among the potential causes. Patients may present during an attack or after the attack has already ended.

Meniere's disease is the prototypical disorder characterized by recurrent spontaneous episodes of dizziness. Patients with this disorder have severe episodes of dizziness—generally true vertigo—with nausea, vomiting, and imbalance.[26] The episodes are accompanied by unilateral auditory features, either hearing loss, a loud "roaring" tinnitus, or severe ear fullness. Episodes are variable in duration but generally will last for hours. The type of tinnitus experienced by patients with Meniere's disease is typically very different from the more common constant bilateral high-pitched tinnitus or the fleeting mild tinnitus that most people experience at some time. The tinnitus in Meniere's disease is usually a very loud roaring sound in one ear. Although the nystagmus may not follow all the rules of peripheral vestibular nystagmus described in vestibular neuritis, the same red flags for central causes (ie, down-beat, pure-torsional, or bidirectional gaze-evoked nystagmus) apply. The head thrust test is generally normal in patients with Meniere's disease since the vestibular nerve is intact.

Transient ischemic attacks (TIA) should be a concern in the patient who presents with new-onset recurrent spontaneous attacks of dizziness. TIA generally lasts for minutes, less than is typical for Meniere's disease. Recurrent spontaneous attacks of dizziness is often the initial symptom of an impending basilar artery occlusion.[7] Transient ischemia should be a leading concern when the patient reports recent onset brief attacks, particularly if the attacks are increasing in frequency (ie, a crescendo pattern). Auditory symptoms can also accompany an ischemic etiology since the anterior inferior cerebellar artery can be involved. As with TIA in general, a CT scan is not helpful for ruling out this cause. CT angiography (CTA) or MR angiography (MRA) are the tests to consider when the integrity of the posterior circulation needs to be assessed.

Other Potential Causes

Migraine is the great mimicker of all causes of dizziness. Symptoms can present as an acute severe attack, positional episodes, or recurrent spontaneous attacks.[27,28] The examination features can suggest a peripheral vestibular or central nervous system localization. As with migraine in general, a strong genetic component is felt to play a role in addition to numerous environmental, food, or lifestyle factors. Patients frequently report that stimuli, such as light, sound, or motion, can trigger or aggravate the symptom. The diagnosis of migraine vertigo, unfortunately, remains a diagnosis of exclusion. Thus, if the symptom is new in onset, diagnoses such as stroke or TIA should still be considered if the features do not fit for a peripheral vestibular disorder. When these causes are excluded, migraine becomes a leading candidate. The main supportive features of this diagnosis are a lack of the key features of the other common disorders, and an onset at least several months before presentation. A headache around the time of the dizziness is frequently reported but is not required. Triptan medicines do not generally improve migraine dizziness symptoms.[29]

Panic disorder is another common cause of dizziness symptoms. Most patients with panic disorder will have the other typical symptoms of panic disorder but the dizziness symptom may be the most bothersome. If a diagnosis of panic disorder is not clear based on the history and physical examination, then a workup may be warranted to exclude the other potential causes.

General medical causes are also common causes of dizziness, although typically true vertigo is not reported. In addition, the finding of nystagmus means that either peripheral or central components of the vestibular system are involved. Thus, nystagmus generally rules out most general medical disorders. A cardiac arrhythmia or myocardial infarction should be considered in the appropriate setting.

MISCONCEPTIONS

A recent physician survey highlights some common misconceptions that exist regarding dizziness presentations.[30] Some physicians feel that the report of "isolated dizziness" can discriminate a stroke etiology from a benign peripheral vestibular disorder. While it is true that the lack of other associated neurologic symptoms reduces the likelihood of stroke diagnosis, numerous reports in literature demonstrate how closely stroke can mimic vestibular neuritis.[3–5] A second misconception is that defining the type of dizziness sensation can be used to discriminate benign from sinister disorders. Some feel that lightheadedness or other vague dizziness sensations make a stroke diagnosis less likely than a report of true vertigo. However, a recent population-based study showed that patients reporting vertigo do not have higher odds of stroke diagnosis than patients reporting "dizziness."[14] A third misconception is that dizziness exacerbated by head motion indicates a benign disorder. The fact is that dizziness from any cause can worsen with head movements. The characteristic of BPPV is that the dizziness symptom is triggered by a head movement, not simply worsened by the movement. Finally, some physicians report that a negative CT scan of the brain rules out stroke. However, a CT scan is an insensitive test for acute stroke, particularly stroke within the posterior fossa.[15–17] Thus, a negative CT scan should not be considered adequate for excluding stroke.

A common theme among these misconceptions is an overreliance on the patient's description of symptoms and an overreliance on CT scans. In this article, most emphasis is placed on the critical components of the examination.

SYMPTOMATIC TREATMENT

Patients who present with severe nausea and vomiting typically require intravenous fluids during the emergency department stay. When drug therapy is necessary to reduce symptoms in the acute setting, generally two different categories of drugs are used: vestibular suppressants and antiemetics. An important point is that medicines to symptomatically reduce dizziness can be effective for acute attacks, but are generally not effective as prophylactic agents. Thus, these medicines are best used during the emergency department visit and not as new daily medicines. When taken on a daily basis, the medicines are more likely to result in side effects or reduce the brain's ability to compensate (as with vestibular neuritis).

The major classes of vestibular suppressants include antihistamines, benzodiazepines, and anticholinergics. Although the exact mechanism of action of these drugs is unclear, most appear to act at the level of the neurotransmitters involved in propagation of impulses from primary to secondary vestibular neurons and in maintenance of tone in the vestibular nuclei. Antiemetic drugs are directed against the areas in the brain controlling vomiting. Dopamine, histamine, acetylcholine, and serotonin are transmitters thought to act on these sites to produce vomiting. Most of the vestibular suppressants have anticholinergics or antihistamine qualities, giving them antiemetic properties in addition to the effects on vertigo. When nausea and vomiting are prominent, a mild vestibular suppressant (such as meclizine) can be combined with an antiemetic (such as prochlorperazine) to control symptoms. These medicines typically have central dopamine antagonist properties and are believed to prevent emesis by inhibition at the chemoreceptor trigger zone. A major side effect of both medicine categories is drowsiness, although this effect probably contributes to the therapeutic effect as well.

Few randomized controlled trials have been conducted on the symptomatic treatment of acute dizziness. In one study, 74 patients were randomized to treatment with either 2 mg of intravenous lorazepam or 50 mg of intravenous dimenhydrinate.[31] The results suggested that dimenhydrinate was more effective for reducing symptoms and improving the ability to ambulate. Dimenhydrinate also resulted in less drowsiness.

SUMMARY

The ability to identify the key features of the three most common benign peripheral vestibular disorders allows the evaluating physician to sort through the most common types of dizziness presentations in the emergency department. The most effective way to "rule-out" a serious cause is to "rule-in" a benign inner ear disorder. When the features are atypical or other red flags appear, sinister causes should be considered. The two presentations with the most at stake are the following: (1) acute severe dizziness when the presentation is atypical for vestibular neuritis, and (2) recurrent attacks of dizziness when the attacks are recent in onset and last only minutes. For these two presentations, an ischemic etiology should be strongly considered even if dizziness is the only symptom and the CT scan is normal. For recurrent positional dizziness, a sinister disorder, such as a structural posterior fossa lesion, should be considered when a central positional pattern of nystagmus is seen or when the patient does not respond to particle repositioning techniques. However, generally central positional nystagmus is caused by disorders that require a less urgent evaluation than acute severe dizziness or recurrent attacks of dizziness.

REFERENCES

1. Burt CW, Schappert SM. Ambulatory care visits to physician offices, hospital out-patient departments, and emergency departments: United States, 1999–2000. Vital Health Stat 2004;13(157):1–70.
2. Newman-Toker DE, Cannon LM, Stofferahn ME, et al. Imprecision in patient reports of dizziness symptom quality: a cross-sectional study conducted in an acute care setting. Mayo Clin Proc 2007;82(11):1329–40.
3. Norrving B, Magnusson M, Holtas S. Isolated acute vertigo in the elderly: vestibular or vascular disease? Acta Neurol Scand 1995;91(1):43–8.
4. Lee H, Cho YW. A case of isolated nodulus infarction presenting as a vestibular neuritis. J Neurol Sci 2004;221(1–2):117–9.
5. Lee H, Sohn SI, Cho YW, et al. Cerebellar infarction presenting isolated vertigo: frequency and vascular topographical patterns. Neurology 2006;67(7): 1178–83.
6. Bertholon P, Bronstein AM, Davies RA, et al. Positional down beating nystagmus in 50 patients: cerebellar disorders and possible anterior semicircular canalithiasis. J Neurol Neurosurg Psychiatr 2002;72(3):366–72.
7. von Campe G, Regli F, Bogousslavsky J. Heralding manifestations of basilar artery occlusion with lethal or severe stroke. J Neurol Neurosurg Psychiatr 2003;74(12):1621–6.
8. Savitz SI, Caplan LR, Edlow JA. Pitfalls in the diagnosis of cerebellar infarction. Acad Emerg Med 2007;14(1):63–8.
9. Baloh RW. Clinical practice. Vestibular neuritis. N Engl J Med 2003;348(11): 1027–32.
10. Baloh RW, Honrubia V. Clinical neurophysiology of the vestibular system. 3rd edition. New York: Oxford University Press; 2001.
11. Halmagyi GM, Curthoys IS. A clinical sign of canal paresis. Arch Neurol 1988; 45(7):737–9.
12. Lewis RF, Carey JP. Images in clinical medicine. Abnormal eye movements associated with unilateral loss of vestibular function. N Engl J Med 2006; 355(24):e26.
13. Kleindorfer DO, Miller R, Moomaw CJ, et al. Designing a message for public education regarding stroke: does FAST capture enough stroke? Stroke 2007; 38(10):2864–8.
14. Kerber KA, Brown DL, Lisabeth LD, et al. Stroke among patients with dizziness, vertigo, and imbalance in the emergency department: a population-based study. Stroke 2006;37(10):2484–7.
15. Chalela JA, Kidwell CS, Nentwich LM, et al. Magnetic resonance imaging and computed tomography in emergency assessment of patients with suspected acute stroke: a prospective comparison. Lancet 2007;369(9558):293–8.
16. Simmons Z, Biller J, Adams HP Jr, et al. Cerebellar infarction: comparison of computed tomography and magnetic resonance imaging. Ann Neurol 1986;19(3): 291–3.
17. Wasay M, Dubey N, Bakshi R. Dizziness and yield of emergency head CT scan: is it cost effective? Emerg Med J 2005;22(4):312.
18. Oppenheim C, Stanescu R, Dormont D, et al. False-negative diffusion-weighted MR findings in acute ischemic stroke. AJNR Am J Neuroradiol 2000;21(8): 1434–40.
19. Strupp M, Zingler VC, Arbusow V, et al. Methylprednisolone, valacyclovir, or the combination for vestibular neuritis. N Engl J Med 2004;351(4):354–61.

20. Strupp M, Arbusow V, Maag KP, et al. Vestibular exercises improve central vestibulospinal compensation after vestibular neuritis. Neurology 1998;51(3): 838–44.

21. Furman JM, Cass SP. Benign paroxysmal positional vertigo. N Engl J Med 1999; 341(21):1590–6.

22. Aw ST, Todd MJ, Aw GE, et al. Benign positional nystagmus: a study of its three-dimensional spatio-temporal characteristics. Neurology 2005;64(11):1897–905.

23. Epley JM. The canalith repositioning procedure: for treatment of benign paroxysmal positional vertigo. Otolaryngol Head Neck Surg 1992;107(3):399–404.

24. Lempert T, Tiel-Wilck K. A positional maneuver for treatment of horizontal-canal benign positional vertigo. Laryngoscope 1996;106(4):476–8.

25. Vannucchi P, Giannoni B, Pagnini P. Treatment of horizontal semicircular canal benign paroxysmal positional vertigo. J Vestib Res 1997;7(1):1–6.

26. Minor LB, Schessel DA, Carey JP. Meniere's disease. Curr Opin Neurol 2004; 17(1):9–16.

27. Dieterich M, Brandt T. Episodic vertigo related to migraine (90 cases): vestibular migraine? J Neurol 1999;246(10):883–92.

28. von Brevern M, Zeise D, Neuhauser H, et al. Acute migrainous vertigo: clinical and oculographic findings. Brain 2005;128(Pt 2):365–74.

29. Neuhauser H, Radtke A, von Brevern M, et al. Zolmitriptan for treatment of migrainous vertigo: a pilot randomized placebo-controlled trial. Neurology 2003;60(5):882–3.

30. Stanton VA, Hsieh YH, Camargo CA Jr, et al. Overreliance on symptom quality in diagnosing dizziness: results of a multicenter survey of emergency physicians. Mayo Clin Proc 2007;82(11):1319–28.

31. Marill KA, Walsh MJ, Nelson BK. Intravenous Lorazepam versus dimenhydrate for treatment of vertigo in the emergency department: a randomized clinical trial. Ann Emerg Med 2000;36(4):310–9.

Management of Transient Ischemia Attacks in the Twenty-First Century

Michael Ross, MD[a],*, Fadi Nahab, MD[b]

KEYWORDS

• Transient ischemic attack • Stroke • Management

The classic definition of a transient ischemic attack (TIA) is a sudden, focal, neurologic deficit resulting from ischemia to the brain or retina lasting less than 24 hours.[1] Although the 24-hour time frame was arbitrarily established, it is clear that most TIA symptoms last less than 1 hour, and typically less than 30 minutes.[2] In 2002, the TIA Working Group redefined TIA as "a brief episode of neurologic dysfunction caused by focal brain or retinal ischemia, with clinical symptoms typically lasting less than one hour, and without evidence of acute infarction."[3] This definition incorporated the use of neuroimaging and suggested that neurologic symptoms of any duration with evidence of a new lesion on neuroimaging should be defined as a stroke.

INITIAL EMERGENCY DEPARTMENT EVALUATION OF PATIENTS WHO HAVE A TRANSIENT ISCHEMIC ATTACK

There are an estimated 800,000 acute strokes per year in the United States, and approximately 15% to 30% are preceded by a TIA.[4,5] The emergency department (ED) is the point of first contact for many patients who have a TIA. There are several important points to consider in their initial evaluation.

When obtaining a history from patients experiencing a TIA, several details are important to consider. This includes the patient's age; the duration of symptoms (specifically if symptoms lasted less than 10 minutes, between 10 and 60 minutes, or greater than 60 minutes); the types of symptoms (specifically, if motor weakness or speech impairment occurred); whether symptoms occurred once or several times in the recent past; the presence of headache or head trauma; a history of diabetes, hypertension, atrial

[a] Department of Emergency Medicine, Emory University, 531 Asbury Circle–Annex, Suite N340, Atlanta, Georgia 30322, USA
[b] Department of Neurology, Emory University, 101 Woodruff Circle, Atlanta, Georgia 30322, USA
* Corresponding author.
E-mail address: maross@emory.edu (M. Ross).

Emerg Med Clin N Am 27 (2009) 51–69
doi:10.1016/j.emc.2008.08.008
0733-8627/08/$ – see front matter © 2009 Elsevier Inc. All rights reserved.

emed.theclinics.com

fibrillation, cancer, a known source of cardioembolism (eg, mural thrombus, carotid stenosis, patent foramen ovale), or a hypercoagulable disorder.

The purpose of physical examination in patients suspected of having a TIA is primarily to exclude the presence of subtle persistent neurologic deficits. A discussion of the stroke physical examination is beyond the scope of this review, but an excellent frame of reference for the stroke examination can be obtained through evaluation of a patient's National Institute of Health Stroke Scale (NIHSS) score. NIHSS training is free and is available online.[6] This training focuses on those aspects of the neurologic examination that are most significant and correspond with thrombolytic treatment eligibility.

Patients who have a TIA should have electrocardiography (ECG) to identify the presence of atrial fibrillation or findings suggestive of conditions associated with a mural thrombus (eg, left ventricular aneurism, dilated cardiomyopathy). Continuous cardiac monitoring may detect paroxysmal atrial fibrillation. Routine ED blood work may include fingerstick glucose level, complete serum chemistry studies, complete blood cell count with platelet count, urinalysis, and coagulation profile (prothrombin time, international normalized ratio, and activated partial thromboplastin time). The primary benefit of the coagulation profile is as baseline laboratory values should the patient go on to develop a stroke that is eligible for thrombolytic therapy, which requires a normal baseline profile. Patients at risk for temporal arteritis should have a sedimentation rate performed. Patients who have a TIA require brain imaging, with CT or MRI, to detect acute stroke. Perhaps more importantly, imaging can detect other pathologic findings, such as intracranial hemorrhage, intracranial masses (eg, tumors), and hydrocephalus. These may act as TIA mimics, and their management is quite different.

From this basic screening information obtained, decisions regarding further management may be made.

CLINICAL RISK SCORES

Patients who have a TIA are at increased risk for a subsequent stroke, with the risk varying among populations. A prospective study of patients who had a TIA diagnosed in the EDs of 16 sites in the Northern California Kaiser-Permanente health maintenance system found that 5% of patients had a stroke within 48 hours and 10.5% of patients had a stroke within 90 days of the TIA.[7] Another prospective study of patients diagnosed with TIA from nine general practices in Oxfordshire, England reported that the risk for stroke was 8% at 7 days, 11.5% at 1 month, and 17.3% at 3 months after a TIA.[8] A multicenter observational study of 1380 patients who had a TIA and were hospitalized in southwest Germany reported an incidence of stroke after a TIA to be 8% during hospitalization (median stay of 10 days).[9] Review of a Canadian stroke registry found that the stroke risk at 30 days after a first TIA was 8%, with half of these strokes occurring within the first 2 days.[10] Because of the variability in risk for stroke among patients who have a TIA, determining the short-term risk for stroke in the individual patient can guide decisions on hospitalization, antithrombotic therapy, and other interventions.

In managing patients who have a TIA, it would be useful to know a given patient's risk for having a stroke in the near future (eg, next 2 days, 7 days, 1 month, 3 months). It would also be useful to be able to determine this risk based on readily available screening information obtained in the ED. Currently, there are three TIA clinical risk stratification scores that have been developed and validated: the California score, the ABCD score, and a hybrid of these two called the ABCD^2 score (**Table 1**).[7,11,12] The California score was derived from a cohort analysis of 1707 patients in a large

Table 1
Point assignment and odds (or hazard) ratios for stroke after transient ischemic attack in three risk scores

Clinical Feature	Points	2 Days	7 Days[a]	90 Days
California				
Age older than 60 years	1	—	—	1.8
Diabetes	1	—	—	2.0
TIA duration >10 minutes	1	—	—	2.3
Weakness with TIA	1	—	—	1.9
Speech impairment with TIA	1	—	—	1.5
ABCD				
Age older than 60 years	1	—	2.57[a]	—
Blood pressure elevation (initial systolic blood pressure >140 mm Hg or diastolic blood pressure >90 mm Hg)	1	—	9.67[a]	—
Clinical feature: unilateral weakness	2	—	6.61[a]	—
Clinical feature: speech disturbance without weakness	1	—	2.59[a]	—
Duration of symptoms 10–60 minutes	1	—	3.08[a]	—
Duration of symptoms >60 minutes	2	—	6.17[a]	—
ABCD^2				
Age older than 60 years	1	1.4	1.4	1.5
Blood pressure elevation (systolic blood pressure >140 mm Hg or diastolic blood pressure >90 mm Hg)	1	2.1	1.9	1.6
Clinical feature: unilateral weakness	2	2.9	3.5	3.2
Clinical feature: speech disturbance without weakness	1	1.4	1.5	1.7
Duration of symptoms 10–60 minutes	1	2	1.9	1.7
Duration of symptoms >60 minutes	2	2.3	2.6	2.1
Diabetes	1	1.6	1.4	1.7

[a] Oxfordshire data reported as hazard ratios; all other data reported as odds ratios.
Data from Refs.[7,11,12]

health maintenance organization who were seen by emergency physicians and given a diagnosis of TIA.[7] Patients were seen at 16 hospitals over 1 year, and five variables were found to be independently predictive of stroke: age older than 60 years (odds ratio [OR] = 1.8); symptoms of weakness (OR = 1.9); symptoms of speech impairment, including dysarthria or aphasia (OR = 1.5); diabetes (OR = 2.0); and symptom duration greater than 10 minutes (OR = 2.3). In patients with no risk factors, no strokes occurred at 90 days; for patients with all five risk factors, 34% experienced a stroke and approximately half of the strokes occurred within the first 48 hours after presentation (**Table 2**).

Table 2
Frequency (percent) of stroke after transient ischemic attack using three risk scores

Risk Score	Points	2 Days	7 Days	90 Days
California				
	0	—	—	0
	1	—	—	3
	2	—	—	7
	3	—	—	11
	4	—	—	15
	5	—	—	34
ABCD				
	0	—	0.0	—
	1	—	0.0	—
	2	—	0.0	—
	3	—	0.0	—
	4	—	2.2	—
	5	—	16.3	—
	6	—	35.5	—
ABCD^2				
Low	0–3	1.0	1.2	3.1
Moderate	4–5	4.1	5.9	9.8
High	6–7	8.1	11.7	17.8

Data from Dyken MI, Conneally M, Haerer AF, et al. Cooperative study of hospital frequency and character of transient ischemic attacks, I: background, organization and clinical surgery. JAMA 1977;237:882–6.

The ABCD score was developed in 2005 to predict the 7-day risk for stroke in patients who have a TIA.[11] The score was initially derived from a cohort of 209 patients who had a TIA and has since been validated in 190 patients and tested for clinical utility in 588 additional patients. The score is composed of the following variables: age older than 60 years (hazard ratio [HR] = 2.6); elevated blood pressure, defined as presenting systolic blood pressure greater than 140 mm Hg or diastolic blood pressure greater than 90 mm Hg (HR = 9.7); clinical features of unilateral weakness (HR = 6.6) or speech disturbance without weakness (HR = 2.6); and duration of symptoms classified as less than 10 minutes (HR = 1.0), 10 to 60 minutes (HR = 3.1), or greater than 60 minutes (HR = 6.2). In the validation study, no patients with an ABCD score of 3 or less experienced a stroke within 1 week, whereas scores greater than 3 were associated with an increased risk for stroke (see **Table 2**).

The developers of the California score and the ABCD score subsequently combined their data, standardized patient selection methods and definitions, and reanalyzed the combined data to derive a unified optimal risk score.[12] The combined cohort included 1916 patients from the original ABCD and California score cohorts, with validation performed in 2893 patients from four independent TIA populations. These results led to the ABCD^2 score, which included a history of diabetes as an additional variable. Prognostic values based on C-statistics improved with the ABCD^2 score compared with the prior scores. In the validation cohort, the ABCD^2 score performed well (C-statistics from 0.62 to 0.83 across cohorts and risk periods of 2, 7, or 90 days). Overall, 21% (n = 1012) of patients were classified as high risk (score: 6–7) with an

8.1% 2-day stroke risk, 45% (n = 2169) as moderate risk (score: 4–5) with a 4.1% 2-day risk, and 34% (n =1628) as low risk (score: 0–3) with a 1.0% 2-day risk (**Fig. 1**; see **Table 2**). The $ABCD^2$ score has since been validated in a retrospective record review assessing the ABCD and $ABCD^2$ scores in 226 patients who had a TIA in Greece, and it was found that both scores were highly predictive of stroke, with the $ABCD^2$ score performing slightly better than the ABCD score (C-statistic for 7-day stroke risk: $ABCD^2$ = 0.80, ABCD = 0.77).[13,14]

Although these clinical risk scores effectively identify those patients at highest risk for subsequent stroke, their ability to identify patients needing emergent treatment has not been established. In one study of 117 patients who had an acute TIA at a single center, the ABCD score performed poorly in identifying patients with large vessel stenosis, cardioembolism, or subsequent stroke or death.[15] These findings emphasize that risk scores should supplement but not replace clinical judgment in the assessment of individual patients. The use of additional data, including neuroimaging (for evaluation of large vessel stenosis), ECG (for atrial fibrillation), and clinical features suggestive of unusual causes of stroke (eg, dissection, endocarditis) may indicate a significant short-term risk for stroke regardless of risk score.

MRI IN TRANSIENT ISCHEMIC ATTACK

In the evaluation of patients who have a TIA, MRI has significant advantages over CT in that it is more sensitive for acute infarcts, and thus can distinguish stroke from TIA, and it is better in the detection of other pathologic findings. MRI should be ordered with gadolinium contrast to increase the sensitivity for blood-brain barrier breakdown, which can be seen with mass lesions or inflammatory processes. MRI diffusion-weighted imaging (DWI) is sensitive for acute ischemic injury. Limitations to the use of MRI include availability, cost, patient tolerance (claustrophobia and metal implants), and time needed for the evaluation. If these limitations were to be overcome, however, it could become the imaging modality of choice for patients who have a stroke and TIA.

The use of DWI MRI sequences can establish the presence of cerebrovascular ischemia in 16% to 67% of patients who have a TIA.[16] Patients who have a TIA with

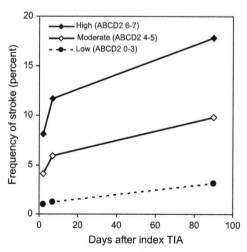

Fig. 1. Risk for stroke after TIA stratified by $ABCD^2$ score strata.

a DWI lesion may represent a higher risk group for subsequent stroke. In one study of 83 patients who had a TIA, the presence of a DWI lesion doubled the risk for a subsequent vascular event. In patients who had a DWI lesion and symptoms lasting longer than 1 hour, the risk was increased fourfold.[17] Another study included 120 patients who had a TIA or minor stroke evaluated within 12 hours of symptom onset and found a 90-day stroke rate in DWI-negative patients of 4.2% and in DWI-positive patients of 14.7% ($P = .10$).[18] Interestingly, patients with negative DWI were 4.6 times more likely to present with a recurrent TIA and 4.3 times less likely to present with a stroke than patients with a DWI lesion.[19]

In addition to the increased risk for subsequent stroke, patients who have a TIA with DWI lesions may also be at greater risk for having high-risk mechanisms, such as high-grade large vessel stenosis or a cardioembolic source. A study of 61 patients who had a TIA found that less than 10% of DWI-negative patients had a high-risk mechanism identified, compared with 60% of DWI-positive patients ($P<.001$).[15] A meta-analysis of 19 studies that examined DWI in patients who had a TIA found that a DWI lesion was associated with the presence of atrial fibrillation (OR = 2.75, 95% confidence interval [CI]: 1.78–4.25; $P<.001$) and ipsilateral carotid stenosis (OR = 1.93, 95% CI: 1.34–2.76; $P = .001$).[20] This study also found that the presence of DWI lesions was associated with symptom duration longer than 1 hour, speech abnormalities (aphasia or dysarthria), and motor weakness. Age and history of hypertension or diabetes were not associated with DWI lesions, suggesting that the relation between the clinical risk scores and the presence of DWI lesions remains uncertain.[15,20] One study that included 203 patients who had an acute TIA has shown that the presence of a DWI lesion independently predicts the risk for subsequent stroke, even after adjusting for ABCD score.[21] On multivariable analysis, an ABCD score of 5 or greater was associated with an HR of 5.0 (95% CI: 1.0–25.8; $P = .06$) and the presence of a DWI lesion was associated with an HR of 10.3 (95% CI: 1.2–86.7; $P = .03$) for subsequent stroke. Larger studies evaluating the role of DWI for predicting subsequent stroke risk are clearly warranted.

VASCULAR IMAGING

TIA associated with large vessel disease seems to be associated with a high short-term risk for stroke. A retrospective subgroup analysis of 603 patients enrolled in the North American Symptomatic Carotid Endarterectomy Trial (NASCET) trial with carotid disease and a hemispheric TIA demonstrated a 90-day stroke risk of 20.1%, with most of this risk accruing within the first 20 days after the index TIA.[22] Although this analysis did not include a matched subgroup without carotid disease, the observed stroke rate was considerably higher than that reported in other studies of unselected patients who had a TIA. In another study, 345 patients who had a TIA within 24 hours of symptom onset underwent carotid and transcranial ultrasonography to identify large vessel disease. On multivariable analysis (including adjustment for ABCD score) the only independent predictor of stroke risk within 7 days was the presence of large vessel occlusive disease (HR = 5.9, 95% CI: 2.2–15.9).[23]

TIA associated with intracranial large vessel disease may also be associated with a high short-term risk for stroke. In a series of 120 patients who had a TIA or minor stroke and underwent magnetic resonance angiography (MRA) of the brain within 12 hours of symptom onset, 12.5% of patients had an intracranial vessel occlusion (all of whom also had a DWI abnormality).[18] The 90-day stroke rate in patients with intracranial vessel occlusion was 32.6%, compared with 10.8% for those with a DWI lesion but no vessel occlusion and 4.3% in patients with no DWI lesion and no vessel occlusion. It is important to note that these patients were not evaluated for evidence of extracranial carotid disease, which may have also been present in patients who had intracranial disease.

Carotid vascular imaging may be obtained using carotid artery duplex ultrasonography, MRI/MRA, and CT angiography. All may be acceptable, with advantages and disadvantages to each, which are listed in **Table 3**.

ECHOCARDIOGRAPHY

TIA practice guidelines recommend that an echocardiogram be obtained in younger patients without a large vessel cause.[24] The purpose is to detect intramural clot in the atria (atrial fibrillation), clot in the ventricle (left ventricle [LV] aneurism or dilated cardiomyopathy with left ventricle ejection fraction [LVEF] <20%), major valvular disease prone to forming emboli (eg, endocarditis, severe mitral stenosis), or a patent foramen ovale associated with a hypercoagulable disorder. Based on probabilities of large vessel disease, the likelihood that a finding would have an impact on therapeutic decision making is inversely proportional to age. Thus, patients younger than 45 years of age are more likely to benefit. Optimal selection criteria for echocardiography in TIA have not been clearly established, however. In general, transthoracic echocardiography is adequate for evaluation of most patients. Transesophageal echocardiography

Table 3
Advantages and disadvantages of various vascular imaging modalities in the evaluation of patients with transient ischemic attack

Imaging Modality	Advantages	Disadvantages
Carotid artery duplex ultrasound	• Present screening standard • Lowest cost • No radiation/contrast	• Need an accredited vascular laboratory • Timeliness of availability • No associated brain imaging • Clarity of report information • Does not identify carotid dissection
CT angiography of head/neck	• May be coupled with initial head CT • Fast • Potential 24-hour availability • Accurate vascular imaging • Imaging of head and neck vessels • May provide perfusion information	• Higher cost • Contrast/renal failure issues • Much more radiation • Limited evidence to support as an alternative to Doppler • More "back-end" reformatting work involved
MRI/MRA of head/neck	• May be coupled with brain MRI (superior brain imaging) • May be done if Doppler or CT angiography is not available • Imaging of head and neck vessels • Provides perfusion information	• Higher cost • Longer imaging acquisition time: more "front-end" work involved • Patient tolerance issues: metal implants/claustrophobia • Timeliness of availability • Contrast/renal failure issues (may be done without if needed)

is more sensitive in identifying clot in the left atrial appendage, which occurs in patients with atrial fibrillation.

INPATIENT VS. OUTPATIENT EVALUATION OF TRANSIENT ISCHEMIC ATTACK

A major challenge facing the emergency physician is to determine which patients who have a TIA should be hospitalized. On the one hand, hospitalization may expedite diagnostic evaluation, hastening identification and intervention for specific high-risk causes of TIA (eg, carotid stenosis, atrial fibrillation). Further, hospitalized patients who have a stroke after a TIA may receive expedited thrombolysis. In a cost-utility analysis, hospitalization for 24 hours had a cost-effectiveness ratio of $55,044 per quality-adjusted life-year purely on the basis of allowing the rapid administration of thrombolytic therapy.[25] Conversely, most patients who have a TIA have a low short-term risk for stroke, and given the expense and resource use associated with admission, the benefit is uncertain.

Currently, there are limited data on the benefit of hospitalization for patients who have a TIA. In a prospective population-based stroke surveillance study over a 5-year period, 552 TIAs were identified and 69% of these patients were hospitalized. The risk for stroke at 30 days was 2% in those hospitalized compared with 7% in those discharged ($P = .002$).[26] Based on two single-center studies (n = 117 and n = 203) that included patients who had a TIA and were admitted to stroke units, the 90-day stroke rates were 1.7% and 3.5%, respectively, which are lower than expected rates (based on ABCD scores).[15,21] It remains unclear if hospitalization may benefit patients by providing an expedited evaluation or through other management differences.

Current guidelines on the need for hospitalization vary widely. The National Stroke Association TIA guidelines published in 2006 recommended that hospitalization be "considered" for patients presenting with a first TIA within the past 24 to 48 hours and be "generally recommended" for patients who have crescendo TIAs, duration of symptoms greater than 1 hour, symptomatic carotid stenosis greater than 50%, a known cardiac source of embolus, a known hypercoagulable state, or an appropriate combination of the California score or ABCD score.[24] The option of outpatient evaluation within 24 to 48 hours in a specialized TIA clinic was also recommended.

Two studies have recently been published advocating the use of urgent-access specialized TIA clinics. In the Early Use of Existing Strategies for Stroke (EXPRESS) study, the use of a rapid-access TIA clinic that included immediate diagnostic testing and treatment initiation was compared with standard outpatient evaluation.[27] This study was nested within an ongoing population-based incidence study of TIA and stroke, the Oxford Vascular Study, and therefore ensured complete case ascertainment and follow-up. In the initial phase of the study, before implementation of the TIA clinic, the rate of stroke at 90 days was 10.3% (32 of 210 patients). After implementation, the stroke rate decreased to 2.1% (6 of 281 patients; $P = .0001$).[27] In another study, 1085 patients who were suspected of having a TIA were evaluated in a hospital-based clinic with around-the-clock access for patients who had a TIA over a 2-year period.[28] The 90-day stroke rate was 1.24% compared with a predicted stroke rate based on patient $ABCD^2$ scores of almost 6%.

In the United States, urgent neurologic evaluation and diagnostic testing can be challenging to arrange on an outpatient basis because of multiple logistic barriers, including scheduling limitations and insurance approval requirements, with suboptimal results achieved in clinical practice. In one study of 95 patients in the United States who presented to their primary care physician with a first TIA, only 23% underwent a brain imaging study, 40% underwent carotid imaging, 18% underwent ECG, and

19% underwent echocardiography.[29] Overall, 31% had no evaluations within the first month of the index visit beyond an examination in the office, and less than half of patients who had a TIA and a history of atrial fibrillation were placed on anticoagulants.

Another option is the use of an observation unit, often in the ED, to carry out an accelerated diagnostic protocol (ADP). This approach has been developed for ED patients with chest pain at low to intermediate risk for acute cardiac ischemia. In a 2003 survey, such units were present in almost 20% of hospitals.[30] Relative to traditional inpatient care, ED ADPs for chest pain have been shown to decrease length of stay and cost and to improve patient satisfaction and quality of life, with comparable diagnostic outcomes.[31,32]

In 2007, Ross and colleagues[33] reported a prospective randomized study of 149 patients who had a TIA and were randomized to inpatient admission (control group) or ED observation unit admission for management using a TIA ADP. All patients who had a TIA had normal findings on CT of the head, ECG, and laboratory studies and had no known embolic source. Both groups had orders for serial clinical examinations, a neurology consult, carotid Doppler ultrasonography, echocardiography, and cardiac monitoring. Patients undergoing the ADP with positive testing were admitted. Compared with the inpatient control group, patients in the ADP group had total length of stays that were half as long (26 vs. 61 hours), lower 90-day total direct costs ($890 vs. $1547), and comparable 90-day clinical outcomes. All positive ADP patient outcomes were identified in the ED, with 15% of patients subsequently admitted as a result of positive ADP outcomes. In this protocol-driven model, more patients undergoing the ADP underwent carotid imaging (97% vs. 90%) and in less time (median: 13 vs. 25 hours) and more ADP patients underwent echocardiography (97% vs. 73%) in less time (median: 19 vs. 43 hours). Both groups had comparable rates of related return visits (12% each), subsequent strokes (three vs. two strokes), and major clinical events (four each). This approach offers a promising alternative to inpatient admission for patients who have a TIA but requires a commitment of resources. Further refinements using alternative imaging and risk stratification tools may increase the utility of this strategy.

ACUTE MANAGEMENT OF TRANSIENT ISCHEMIC ATTACK

The goal of initial management of patients who have a TIA is to optimize potentially compromised cerebral blood flow. This includes positioning the patient with the head of the bed flat, permissive hypertension, and administration of intravenous fluids. A study of 69 patients who had an acute TIA using perfusion MRI found that one third of patients had evidence of a perfusion abnormality.[34] Simply changing head position has been shown to increase cerebral perfusion in studies using transcranial Doppler monitoring. The mean flow velocity in the middle cerebral artery can increase 20% when head position is lowered from 30° to 0°.[35]

Another simple intervention is called "permissive hypertension." This is the avoidance of blood pressure–lowering agents. The basis for this treatment is that during acute cerebrovascular ischemia, cerebral autoregulation may be impaired and cerebral perfusion in regions that depend on collateral blood flow may depend on systemic blood pressure. This was confirmed in a controlled trial of nimodipine in acute ischemic stroke, which found that poor outcomes in nimodipine-treated patients were associated with blood pressure lowering.[36] Other studies have identified that early blood pressure lowering is a predictor of poor outcome after stroke.[37] Careful administration of isotonic intravenous fluids can ensure euvolemia and maintain intravascular volume.

In patients who have a confirmed TIA, without intracranial hemorrhage, antithrombotic therapy should be started as soon as possible. Presently, there are limited data from randomized trials involving treatment of patients who have a TIA in the first 24 to 48 hours after symptom onset. More data exist for ischemic stroke, a group whose risk for intracranial hemorrhage might be higher because of brain tissue infarction and whose risk for subsequent stroke is lower than that of patients who have a TIA. Because of this, the risk may be lower and the benefit greater for initiation of antithrombotic therapy in patients who have a TIA. Some of these benefits may be extrapolated from stroke studies to patients who have a TIA.[22,38–40]

Antiplatelet Therapy

The International Stroke Trial (IST) and the Chinese Acute Stroke Trial (CAST) have evaluated the role of early aspirin therapy in acute ischemic stroke. The IST randomized 19,435 patients to aspirin at a dosage of 300 mg/d or no aspirin, with treatment started within 48 hours of symptom onset.[41] Treatment with aspirin reduced the rate of recurrent ischemic stroke from 3.9% to 2.8% ($P<.05$) and showed a trend toward reduced mortality (9.0% vs. 9.4%) at 2 weeks or by hospital discharge. There was no significant difference in intracranial bleeding between the two groups. The CAST randomized 21,106 patients to aspirin at a dosage of 160 mg/d or placebo within 48 hours of symptom onset.[42] Treatment with aspirin reduced the rate of recurrent ischemic stroke from 2.1% to 1.6% ($P = .01$) and mortality from 3.9% to 3.3% ($P = .04$) at 4 weeks or by hospital discharge. There was a trend toward excess intracranial bleeding with aspirin (1.1% vs. 0.9%). A pooled analysis of the IST and CAST showed that aspirin treatment reduced recurrent ischemic stroke by 7 per 1000 patients treated ($P<.0001$) and reduced mortality by a further 4 per 1000 patients treated ($P = .05$). Aspirin did result in a small increase in intracranial bleeding of 2 per 1000 patients treated ($P = .07$), however.[43]

The combination of aspirin and clopidogrel was recently evaluated in the Fast Assessment of Stroke and Transient Ischemic Attack to Prevent Early Recurrence (FASTER) study.[44] In this study, 392 patients who had a high-risk TIA or minor stroke were randomized within 24 hours of symptom onset to aspirin alone vs. aspirin and clopidogrel; patients were also randomized to simvastatin vs. placebo in a 2×2 factorial design. Compared with aspirin alone, the combination of aspirin and clopidogrel was associated with a trend toward reduction in the primary end point of stroke within 90 days (7.1% vs. 10.8%; $P = .19$). As expected, most events occurred early in the trial, with a median time to stroke end point of 1 day. An excess of symptomatic bleeding events was seen with combination therapy (3.0% vs. 0%; $P = .03$). Confirmatory trials are planned.

Anticoagulation

Several randomized controlled trials have evaluated the role of early anticoagulation in patients who have an ischemic stroke. Unfortunately, there are limited data on the role of early anticoagulation in patients who have a TIA.[45–47] Berge and Sandercock[48] performed a meta-analysis of several trials evaluating heparin or low-molecular-weight heparin and found there to be no net benefit of early anticoagulation in ischemic stroke. It remains uncertain whether patients who have a TIA may benefit from early anticoagulation because of their lower risk for hemorrhage and increased risk for recurrent stroke when compared with patients who have an ischemic stroke, however.

Thrombolysis for Post-Transient Ischemic Attack Stroke

Patients who develop stroke after a TIA are eligible for thrombolytic therapy. Pooled data from randomized controlled trials have demonstrated that thrombolytic therapy for acute ischemic stroke is critically time dependent, with earlier treatment associated with better outcomes.[49] Close neurologic observation in the ED or hospital setting may therefore allow expedited thrombolysis should a stroke occur after a TIA.

INTERMEDIATE AND LONG-TERM STROKE PREVENTION AFTER TRANSIENT ISCHEMIC ATTACK

The optimal prevention strategy in patients who have a TIA requires determination of the underlying mechanism causing the ischemic event. Mechanisms of TIA that have particular relevance to the emergency physician because of direct therapeutic implications include cervical carotid artery stenosis, cardioembolism, carotid or vertebral artery dissection, and infective endocarditis.

Cervical Carotid Stenosis and Carotid Endarterectomy

Patients who have a TIA attributable to carotid stenosis of 70% to 99% benefit from revascularization with carotid endarterectomy to reduce the risk for recurrent stroke. In two large randomized trials, the European Carotid Surgery Trial and the North American Symptomatic Carotid Endarterectomy Trial, patients who had a TIA or nondisabling stroke caused by 70% to 99% carotid stenosis had a 10% to 15% absolute risk reduction in subsequent stroke.[50] Older patients (age >75 years) had a greater incremental benefit in their stroke risk reduction relative to younger patients. A pooled analysis of both trials showed a dramatic benefit when carotid endarterectomy was performed within 2 weeks of the symptomatic event as opposed to a later time point.[50,51] There is a 30.2% absolute risk reduction in the 5-year risk for stroke and operative death if carotid revascularization occurs within 2 weeks of the sentinel event. This benefit drops to 17.6% if surgery is delayed to 2 to 4 weeks and to 11.4% if it is delayed to 4 to 12 weeks. Similar trends are seen in patients who have symptomatic carotid stenosis in the range of 50% to 70%. These data emphasize the need for prompt surgical intervention in these patients, ideally within 2 weeks of their sentinel TIA. With the development of endovascular carotid stenting, there is increasing interdisciplinary competition for patients requiring revascularization among neurosurgeons, vascular surgeons, interventional cardiologists, interventional radiologists, and even interventional neurologists. In some centers, this has changed practice patterns and markedly shortened the interval between TIA and revascularization procedures.

Atrial Fibrillation

Warfarin is substantially more effective than aspirin in the prevention of recurrent stroke in patients who have experienced a TIA or stroke secondary to atrial fibrillation. A meta-analysis of 12 trials, including almost 13,000 patients, found that warfarin was associated with a 39% relative risk reduction (95% CI: 22%–52%) compared with antiplatelet therapy and only a small absolute increased risk for bleeding complications.[52] Combination therapy with aspirin and clopidogrel has been shown to be inferior to warfarin therapy in patients with atrial fibrillation. The Atrial Fibrillation Clopidogrel Trial with Irbesartan for Prevention of Vascular Events (ACTIVE) study randomized 6706 patients to adjusted-dose warfarin or combination therapy with aspirin and clopidogrel.[53] The annual risk for vascular events was 3.9% with warfarin and 5.6% with aspirin and clopidogrel ($P = .0003$), with similar rates of major bleeding between the two groups.

Long-term anticoagulation has clearly been shown to be beneficial in terms of stroke prevention. It remains uncertain whether patients who have a TIA and atrial fibrillation should be treated with parenteral anticoagulant therapy during the acute period, however. It has been shown that relative to aspirin alone, there is no net benefit of parenteral anticoagulation of patients who have an acute ischemic stroke with atrial fibrillation.[41,54] Whether differences in the risk for hemorrhage and the risk for early stroke recurrence between patients who have a TIA vs. a stroke may result in a net benefit for early parenteral anticoagulation remains uncertain.

Carotid or Vertebral Artery Dissection and Anticoagulation

The mural hematoma present in arterial dissection can result in vessel occlusion or can serve as a source of emboli resulting in a TIA or stroke. There have been no randomized trials to assess optimal antithrombotic therapy in arterial dissection. A Cochrane database systematic review of carotid dissection that includes only reported case series found a trend toward improved outcomes with anticoagulation compared with antiplatelet therapy (14.3% vs. 23.7% dead or disabled, OR = 1.94, 95% CI: 0.76–4.91).[55] Recurrent stroke was seen in 1.7% of patients with anticoagulation vs. 3.8% with antiplatelet therapy and 3.3% with no therapy. These data are limited by their nonrandomized nature and the susceptibility to publication bias, leaving the benefit of anticoagulation over antiplatelet therapy in these patients uncertain.

Infectious Endocarditis

Embolic TIA attributable to bacterial endocarditis mandates immediate anti-infective therapy and cardiology evaluation. Given the high risk for intracranial bleeding, intravenous anticoagulation should be avoided in these patients.

Antiplatelet Therapy for Stroke Prevention After Transient Ischemic Attack

The use of antiplatelet therapy in the acute management of TIA was previously discussed, but subacute initiation of antiplatelet therapy for secondary stroke prevention has been studied even more extensively. Several large randomized trials have evaluated the role of antiplatelet therapy for secondary stroke prevention in patients with a history of TIA or ischemic stroke. Antiplatelet therapies currently available include aspirin, the thienopyridines (including clopidogrel and ticlopidine), and the combination of aspirin and extended-release dipyridamole (ER-DP).

Aspirin

Aspirin therapy reduces the risk for recurrent stroke, myocardial infarction, or vascular death by approximately 20% in patients who have had a recent TIA. This translates into 36 events prevented for every 1000 patients treated over a 2.5-year period.[56] Higher dose aspirin (300–1500 mg) is no more effective than low-dose aspirin (50–75 mg) but is associated with a greater incidence of side effects.[56,57]

Thienopyridines (clopidogrel, ticlopidine)

Clopidogrel has been shown to be slightly more effective than aspirin based on results from the Clopidogrel vs. Aspirin in Patients at Risk of Ischemic Events (CAPRIE) study.[58] The relative risk reduction compared with aspirin was small (8.7%) for the primary end points of stroke, myocardial infarction, or vascular death. In the subgroup of patients with a recent history of ischemic stroke (n = 6431), there was a nonsignificant relative risk reduction of 7.3%. Adverse events in the clopidogrel and aspirin groups were similar. Ticlopidine, another thienopyridine agent, has shown conflicting results in clinical trials, and its side effect of severe neutropenia has limited its utility in clinical practice.[59–61]

Combination antiplatelet therapies

Two large randomized studies have shown that the combination of aspirin and ER-DP is more effective than aspirin alone in preventing recurrent stroke in patients with a history of TIA or ischemic stroke. In the European Stroke Prevention Study-2 (ESPS-2) of patients who had a recent stroke or TIA given placebo, aspirin alone, or ER-DP, the combination of aspirin and ER-DP was significantly more effective than either agent alone, with a relative risk reduction of 23% compared with aspirin and no significant increase in major bleeding. Compared with aspirin alone, approximately 30 strokes were prevented for every 1000 patients treated with ER-DP for over 2 years.[62] The European/Australasian Stroke Prevention in Reversible Ischemia Trial (ESPRIT) randomized patients who had a recent stroke or TIA to aspirin or aspirin in combination with dipyridamole.[63] The primary end point was a composite of stroke, myocardial infarction, vascular death, or major bleeding. A significant benefit in favor of combination therapy was demonstrated (HR = 0.80, 95% CI: 0.66–0.98). Approximately 30 events were prevented for every 1000 patients treated over 3.5 years. The most common side effect of combination therapy with aspirin and dipyridamole is headache, caused by the dipyridamole component, which improves after several days of use.

Another two large trials have studied combination therapy with clopidogrel and aspirin, the Management of Atherothrombosis with Clopidogrel in High-Risk Patients (MATCH) trial and the Clopidogrel for High Atherothrombotic Risk and Ischemic Stabilization, Management, and Avoidance (CHARISMA) trial. These studies found no benefit to this combination relative to either drug alone but did find an increase in the risk for bleeding. The results of the MATCH and CHARISMA trials suggest that the combination of clopidogrel and aspirin should be avoided in patients who have isolated cerebrovascular disease.[64,65]

At this time, the largest antiplatelet trial for stroke prevention, the Prevention Regimen for Effectively Avoiding Second Strokes (PRoFESS) trial, has recently been completed with results not yet published.[66] It enrolled more than 20,000 patients to compare the combination of aspirin and ER-DP with clopidogrel in patients with a history of stroke or TIA with imaging evidence of tissue infarction.

Guidelines for antiplatelet therapy for stroke prevention

The American Heart Association/American Stroke Association (AHA/ASA) and American College of Chest Physicians (ACCP) have each published independent guidelines on use of antiplatelet therapy for prevention of recurrent stroke after a stroke or TIA.[67–69] Both recommend the use of antiplatelet therapy for patients who have a noncardioembolic TIA (AHA/ASA: class I, level of evidence A; ACCP: grade I). Aspirin at a dosage of 50 to 325 mg/d; the combination of aspirin, 25 mg, and ER-DP, 200 mg, twice daily; and clopidogrel at a dose of 75 mg/d are all considered acceptable options. Initial therapy with aspirin and ER-DP is suggested instead of aspirin alone (AHA/ASA: class I, level of evidence B; ACCP: grade 2A), and clopidogrel may be considered instead of aspirin alone (AHA/ASA: class IIb, level of evidence B; ACCP grade 2B). The combination of aspirin and clopidogrel is not routinely recommended (AHA/ASA: class III, level of evidence A). The AHA/ASA guidelines emphasize that the selection of antiplatelet agents should be individualized on the basis of patient characteristics, such as risk profile and tolerance of side effects.

OTHER STROKE PREVENTION STRATEGIES

The use of statin medications has been shown to lead to a significant reduction in the 1-year risk for recurrent vascular events in patients who have had a TIA or stroke in large randomized controlled trials.[70–72] Early initiation of statin therapy during hospitalization has been shown to increase long-term compliance and may have a potential neuroprotectant effect.[73–75] Although most vascular neurologists agree that blood pressure should not be lowered in the acute setting after a TIA, it is also evident

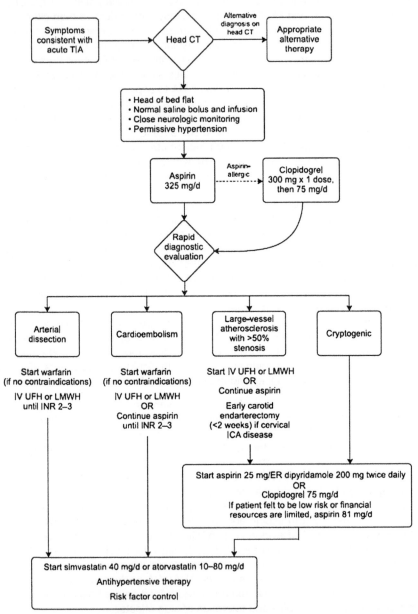

Fig. 2. The flow chart illustrates one approach to the management of patients with a TIA. ICA, internal carotid artery; INR, international normalized ratio; IV, intravenous; LMWH, low-molecular-weight heparin; UFH, unfractionated heparin. (*Adapted from* Cucchiara B, Ross M. Transient ischemic attack: risk stratification and treatment. Ann Emerg Med 2008;52:S27–39; with permission.)

from controlled trials that long-term blood pressure control is an important part of stroke prevention.[76] AHA/ASA guidelines for acute ischemic stroke suggest that antihypertensive treatment in the acute setting be withheld unless the systolic blood pressure exceeds 220 mm Hg or diastolic blood pressure exceeds 120 mm Hg, unless there is another indication for blood pressure lowering (eg, cardiac ischemia, aortic dissection).[77] These guidelines also suggest restarting antihypertensive medications in patients with preexisting hypertension who are neurologically stable after 24 hours. One international guideline suggests waiting 7 to 14 days after a TIA before starting antihypertensive therapy, however.[24] It is important to note that these guidelines are not based on evidence from controlled trials, and ongoing trials should better clarify these recommendations. Other measures, including smoking cessation, control of blood glucose levels in diabetic patients, regular exercise, and healthy eating habits, should also be emphasized.

Fig. 2 summarizes one approach to the management of patients who have a TIA.[78]

SUMMARY

Recognition of the short-term risk for stroke facing patients who have a TIA and the availability of evidence-based treatments for recurrent stroke prevention have brought about an understanding that a TIA should be evaluated and treated with the same urgency applied to patients who have unstable angina. Further research is needed to optimize our ability to risk-stratify patients and to provide further evidence-based treatment options for patients who have a TIA.

REFERENCES

1. Special report from the National Institute of Neurological Disorders and Stroke. Classification of cerebrovascular diseases III. Stroke 1990;21:637–76.
2. Dyken MI, Conneally M, Haerer AF, et al. Cooperative study of hospital frequency and character of transient ischemic attacks, I: background, organization and clinical surgery. JAMA 1977;237:882–6.
3. Albers GW, Caplan LR, Easton JD. Transient ischemic attack—proposal for a new definition. N Engl J Med 2002;347:1713–6.
4. Hankey GJ. Impact of treatment of people with transient ischemic attack on stroke incidence and public health. Cerebrovasc Dis 1996;6(Suppl 1):26–33.
5. Rothwell PM, Warlow CP. Timing of TIAs preceding stroke: time window for prevention is very short. Neurology 2005;64:817–20.
6. Available at: www.nihstrokescale.org or professionaleducationcenter.american heart.org.
7. Johnston SC, Gress DR, Browner WS, et al. Short-term prognosis after emergency department diagnosis of TIA. JAMA 2000;284:2901–6.
8. Coull AJ, Lovett JK, Rothwell PM. Population based study of early risk of stroke after transient ischaemic attack or minor stroke: implications for public education and organisation of services. BMJ 2004;328:326–8.
9. Daffertshofer M, Mielke O, Pullwitt A, et al. Transient ischemic attacks are more than "ministrokes." Stroke 2004;35:2453–8.
10. Gladstone DJ, Kapral MK, Fang J, et al. Management and outcomes of transient ischemic attacks in Ontario. CMAJ 2004;170:1099–104.
11. Rothwell PM, Giles MF, Flossmann E, et al. A simple score (ABCD) to identify individuals at high early risk of stroke after transient ischaemic attack. Lancet 2005;366:29–36.

12. Johnston SC, Rothwell PM, Nguyen-Huynh MN, et al. Validation and refinement of scores to predict very early stroke risk after transient ischaemic attack. Lancet 2007;369:283–92.

13. Tsivgoulis G, Spengos K, Manta P, et al. Validation of the ABCD score in identifying individuals at high early risk of stroke after a transient ischemic attack: a hospital-based case series study. Stroke 2006;37:2892–7.

14. Tsivgoulis G, Vassilopoulou S, Spengos K. Potential applicability of ABCD score in triaging TIA patients. Lancet 2007;369:1082.

15. Cucchiara BL, Messe SR, Taylor RA, et al. Is the ABCD score useful for risk stratification of patients with acute transient ischemic attack? Stroke 2006;37: 1710–4.

16. Redgrave JN, Coutts SB, Schulz UG, et al. Systematic review of associations between the presence of acute ischemic lesions on diffusion-weighted imaging and clinical predictors of early stroke risk after transient ischemic attack. Stroke 2007;38:1482–8.

17. Purroy F, Montaner J, Rovira A, et al. Higher risk of further vascular events among transient ischemic attack patients with diffusion-weighted imaging acute ischemic lesions. Stroke 2004;35:2313–9.

18. Coutts SB, Simon JE, Eliasziw M, et al. Triaging transient ischemic attack and minor stroke patients using acute magnetic resonance imaging. Ann Neurol 2005;57:848–54.

19. Boulanger JM, Coutts SB, Eliasziw M, et al. Diffusion-weighted imaging-negative patients with transient ischemic attack are at risk of recurrent transient events. Stroke 2007;38:2367–9.

20. Redgrave JN, Schulz UG, Briley D, et al. Presence of acute ischaemic lesions on diffusion-weighted imaging is associated with clinical predictors of early risk of stroke after transient ischaemic attack. Cerebrovasc Dis 2007;24:86–90.

21. Calvet D, Lamy C, Touze E, et al. Management and outcome of patients with transient ischemic attack admitted to a stroke unit. Cerebrovasc Dis 2007;24:80–5.

22. Eliasziw M, Kennedy J, Hill MD, et al. Early risk of stroke after a transient ischemic attack in patients with internal carotid artery disease. CMAJ 2004;170:1105–9.

23. Purroy F, Molina CA, Montaner J, et al. Absence of usefulness of ABCD score in the early risk of stroke of transient ischemic attack patients. Stroke 2007;38:855–6 [author reply 857].

24. Johnston SC, Nguyen-Huynh MN, Schwarz ME, et al. National Stroke Association guidelines for the management of transient ischemic attacks. Ann Neurol 2006; 60:301–13.

25. Nguyen-Huynh MN, Johnston SC. Is hospitalization after TIA cost-effective on the basis of treatment with TPA? Neurology 2005;65:1799–801.

26. Poisson SN, Lisabeth LD, Brown DL, et al. Effect of hospital admission on stroke risk following TIA. Neurology 2007;68(Suppl 1):A193.

27. Rothwell PM, Giles MF, Chandratheva A, et al. Early Use of Existing Strategies for Stroke (EXPRESS) study. Effect of urgent treatment of transient ischaemic attack and minor stroke on early recurrent stroke (EXPRESS study): a prospective population-based sequential comparison. Lancet 2007;370:1432–42.

28. Lavallée PC, Mesequer E, Abboud H, et al. A transient ischaemic attack clinic with round-the-clock access (SOS-TIA): feasibility and effects. Lancet Neurol 2007;6:953–60.

29. Goldstein LB, Bian J, Samsa GP, et al. New transient ischemic attack and stroke: outpatient management by primary care physicians. Arch Intern Med 2000;160: 2941–6.

30. Mace SE, Graff L, Mikhail M, et al. A national survey of observation units in the United States. Am J Emerg Med 2003;21:529–33.
31. Roberts RR, Zalenski RJ, Mensah EK, et al. Costs of an emergency department-based accelerated diagnostic protocol vs hospitalization in patients with chest pain: a randomized controlled trial. JAMA 1997;278:1670–6.
32. Gomez MA, Anderson JL, Karagounis LA, et al. An emergency department-based protocol for rapidly ruling out myocardial ischemia reduces hospital time and expense: results of a randomized study (ROMIO). J Am Coll Cardiol 1996; 28:25–33.
33. Ross MA, Compton S, Medado P, et al. An emergency department diagnostic protocol for patients with transient ischemic attack: a randomized controlled trial. Ann Emerg Med 2007;50:109–19.
34. Krol AL, Coutts SB, Simon JE, et al. for the VSG. Perfusion MRI abnormalities in speech or motor transient ischemic attack patients. Stroke 2005;36:2487–9.
35. Wojner-Alexander AW, Garami Z, Chernyshev OY, et al. Heads down: flat positioning improves blood flow velocity in acute ischemic stroke. Neurology 2005; 64:1354–7.
36. Ahmed N, Wahlgren NG. Effects of blood pressure lowering in the acute phase of total anterior circulation infarcts and other stroke subtypes. Cerebrovasc Dis 2003;15:235–43.
37. Oliveira-Filho J, Silva SC, Trabuco CC, et al. Detrimental effect of blood pressure reduction in the first 24 hours of acute stroke onset. Neurology 2003;61:1047–51.
38. Sherman DG, Albers GW, Bladin C, et al. The efficacy and safety of enoxaparin vs. unfractionated heparin for the Prevention of Venous Thromboembolism After Acute Ischaemic Stroke (PREVAIL study): an open-label randomised comparison. Lancet 2007;369:1347–55.
39. Johnston SC, Leira EC, Hansen MD, et al. Early recovery after cerebral ischemia risk of subsequent neurological deterioration. Ann Neurol 2003;54:439–44.
40. Wiebers DO, Whisnant JP, O'Fallon WM. Reversible ischemic neurologic deficit (RIND) in a community: Rochester, Minnesota, 1955–1974. Neurology 1982;32: 459–65.
41. International Stroke Trial Collaborative Group. The International Stroke Trial (IST): a randomised trial of aspirin, heparin, both, or neither among 19435 patients with acute ischaemic stroke. Lancet 1997;349:1569–81.
42. CAST (Chinese Acute Stroke Trial) Collaborative Group. CAST: randomised placebo-controlled trial of early aspirin use in 20,000 patients with acute ischemic stroke. Lancet 1997;349:1641–9.
43. Chen ZM, Sandercock P, Pan HC, et al. Indications for early aspirin use in acute ischemic stroke: a combined analysis of 40,000 randomized patients from the Chinese Acute Stroke Trial and the International Stroke Trial. On behalf of the CAST and IST collaborative groups. Stroke 2000;31:1240–9.
44. Kennedy J, Hill MD, Ryckborst KJ, et al. Fast Assessment of Stroke and Transient Ischemic Attack to Prevent Early Recurrence (FASTER): a randomized controlled pilot trial. Lancet Neurol 2007;6:961–9.
45. Biller J, Bruno A, Adams HP, et al. A randomized trial of aspirin or heparin in hospitalized patients with recent transient ischemic attacks. A pilot study. Stroke 1989;20:441–7.
46. Putnam SF, Adams HP. Usefulness of heparin in initial management of patients with recent transient ischemic attacks. Arch Neurol 1985;42:960–2.
47. Keith DS, Phillips SJ, Whisnant JP, et al. Heparin therapy for recent transient focal cerebral ischemia. Mayo Clin Proc 1987;62:1101–6.

48. Berge E, Sandercock P. Anticoagulants vs. antiplatelet agents for acute ischaemic stroke. Cochrane Database Syst Rev 2002:CD003242.
49. Hacke W, Donnan G, Fieschi C, et al. Association of outcome with early stroke treatment: pooled analysis of ATLANTIS, ECASS, and NINDS rt-PA stroke trials. Lancet 2004;363:768–74.
50. Rothwell PM, Eliasziw M, Gutnikov SA, et al. Endarterectomy for symptomatic carotid stenosis in relation to clinical subgroups and timing of surgery. Lancet 2004;363:915–24.
51. Alamowitch S, Eliasziw M, Algra A, et al. Risk, causes, and prevention of ischaemic stroke in elderly patients with symptomatic internal-carotid-artery stenosis. Lancet 2001;357:1154–60.
52. Hart RG, Pearce LA, Aguilar MI. Meta-analysis: antithrombotic therapy to prevent stroke in patients who have nonvalvular atrial fibrillation. Ann Intern Med 2007; 146:857–67.
53. Connolly S, Pogue J, Hart R, et al. Clopidogrel plus aspirin vs. oral anticoagulation for atrial fibrillation in the Atrial Fibrillation Clopidogrel Trial with Irbesartan for Prevention of Vascular Events (ACTIVE W): a randomised controlled trial. Lancet 2006;367:1903–12.
54. Berge E, Abdelnoor M, Nakstad PH, et al. Low molecular-weight heparin vs. aspirin in patients with acute ischaemic stroke and atrial fibrillation: a double-blind randomised study. HAEST Study Group. Heparin in Acute Embolic Stroke Trial. Lancet 2000;355:1205–10.
55. Lyrer P, Engelter S. Antithrombotic drugs for carotid artery dissection. Cochrane Database Syst Rev 2003:CD000255.
56. Antithrombotic Trialists' Collaboration. Collaborative meta-analysis of randomised trials of antiplatelet therapy for prevention of death, myocardial infarction, and stroke in high risk patients. BMJ 2002;324:71–86.
57. Serebruany VL, Steinhubl SR, Berger PB, et al. Analysis of risk of bleeding complications after different doses of aspirin in 192,036 patients enrolled in 31 randomized controlled trials. Am J Cardiol 2005;95:1218–22.
58. CAPRIE Steering Committee. A randomised, blinded, trial of clopidogrel vs. aspirin in patients at risk of ischaemic events (CAPRIE). Lancet 1996;348: 1329–39.
59. Hass WK, Easton JD, Adams HP, et al. A randomized trial comparing ticlopidine hydrochloride with aspirin for the prevention of stroke in high-risk patients. N Engl J Med 1989;321:501–7.
60. Gent M, Blakely JA, Easton JD, et al. The Canadian American Ticlopidine Study (CATS) in thromboembolic stroke. Lancet 1989;1:1215–20.
61. Gorelick PB, Richardson D, Kelly M, et al. Aspirin and ticlopidine for prevention of recurrent stroke in black patients: a randomized trial. JAMA 2003;289:2947–57.
62. Diener HC, Cunha L, Forbes C, et al. European Stroke Prevention Study 2. Dipyridamole and acetylsalicylic acid in the secondary prevention of stroke. J Neurol Sci 1996;143:1–13.
63. Halkes PH, van Gijn J, Kappelle LJ, et al. Aspirin plus dipyridamole vs. aspirin alone after cerebral ischaemia of arterial origin (ESPRIT): randomised controlled trial. Lancet 2006;367:1665–73.
64. Diener HC, Bogousslavsky J, Brass LM, et al. Aspirin and clopidogrel compared with clopidogrel alone after recent ischaemic stroke or transient ischaemic attack in high-risk patients (MATCH): randomised, double-blind, placebo-controlled trial. Lancet 2004;364:331–7.

65. Bhatt DL, Fox KA, Hacke W, et al. Clopidogrel and aspirin vs. aspirin alone for the prevention of atherothrombotic events. N Engl J Med 2006;354:1706–17.
66. Diener HC, Sacco R, Yusuf S, for Steering Committee and PRoFESS Study Group. Rationale, design and baseline data of a randomized, double-blind, controlled trial comparing two antithrombotic regimens (a fixed-dose combination of extended-release dipyridamole plus ASA with clopidogrel) and telmisartan vs. placebo in patients with strokes: the Prevention Regimen for Effectively Avoiding Second Strokes Trial (PRoFESS). Cerebrovasc Dis 2007;23:368–80.
67. Sacco RL, Adams R, Albers G, et al. Guidelines for prevention of stroke in patients with ischemic stroke or transient ischemic attack: a statement for healthcare professionals from the American Heart Association/American Stroke Association Council on stroke: co-sponsored by the Council on Cardiovascular Radiology and Intervention: the American Academy of Neurology affirms the value of this guideline. Stroke 2006;37:577–617.
68. Albers GW, Amarenco P, Easton JD, et al. Antithrombotic and thrombolytic therapy for ischemic stroke: the Seventh ACCP Conference on Antithrombotic and Thrombolytic Therapy. Chest 2004;126:483S–512S.
69. Adams RJ, Albers G, Alberts MJ, et al. Update to the AHA/ASA recommendations for the prevention of stroke in patients with stroke and transient ischemic attack. Stroke 2008;39:1647–52.
70. Collins R, Armitage J, Parish S, et al. Effects of cholesterol-lowering with simvastatin on stroke and other major vascular events in 20536 people with cerebrovascular disease or other high-risk conditions. Lancet 2004;363:757–67.
71. Amarenco P, Bogousslavsky J, Callahan A III, et al. High-dose atorvastatin after stroke or transient ischemic attack. N Engl J Med 2006;355:549–59.
72. Briel M, Schwartz GG, Thompson PL, et al. Effects of early treatment with statins on short-term clinical outcomes in acute coronary syndromes: a meta-analysis of randomized controlled trials. JAMA 2006;295:2046–56.
73. Aronow HD, Novaro GM, Lauer MS, et al. In-hospital initiation of lipid-lowering therapy after coronary intervention as a predictor of long-term utilization: a propensity analysis. Arch Intern Med 2003;163:2576–82.
74. Cucchiara B, Kasner SE. Use of statins in CNS disorders. J Neurol Sci 2001;187: 81–9.
75. Goldstein LB, Investigators SPARCL. The SPARCL trial: effect of statins on stroke severity. Ann Neurol 2006;60(Suppl 10):S85.
76. Progress Collaborative Group. Randomised trial of a perindopril-based blood-pressure-lowering regimen among 6,105 individuals with previous stroke or transient ischaemic attack. Lancet 2001;358:1033–41.
77. Adams HP Jr, del Zoppo G, Alberts MJ, et al. Guidelines for the early management of adults with ischemic stroke: a guideline from the American Heart Association/American Stroke Association Stroke Council, Clinical Cardiology Council, Cardiovascular Radiology and Intervention Council, and the Atherosclerotic Peripheral Vascular Disease and Quality of Care Outcomes in Research Interdisciplinary Working Groups: the American Academy of Neurology affirms the value of this guideline as an educational tool for neurologists. Circulation 2007;115: e478–534.
78. Cucchiara B, Ross M. Transient ischemic attack: risk stratification and treatment. Ann Emerg Med 2008;52:S27–39.

Diagnosis and Management of the Primary Headache Disorders in the Emergency Department Setting

Benjamin Wolkin Friedman, MD, MS[a],*, Brian Mitchell Grosberg, MD[b]

KEYWORDS

• Headache • Migraine • Emergency department

Headache continues to be a frequent cause of emergency department (ED) use, accounting for 2% of all visits to United States EDs.[1] In these visits, the most commonly diagnosed are the primary headache disorders, most often migraine or tension-type headache.[2–4] The primary headache disorders are a collection of chronic illnesses characterized by repeated acute exacerbations, sometimes warranting an ED visit. The cornerstones of ED management are: (1) to determine the correct headache diagnosis, (2) to exclude secondary causes of headache, such as infection, mass-lesion, or hemorrhage, (3) to initiate headache abortive therapy in appropriate cases, (4) to provide the patient with an appropriate discharge plan that includes a diagnosis, patient education, and prescriptions, and (5) to give prompt referral to an appropriate health care provider for definitive management. This article reviews the diagnosis and management of the primary headache disorders, including migraine, tension-type headache, and cluster. In addition, less common primary headache disorders are reviewed.

Diagnosing or classifying the individual headache can be challenging, but allows appropriate treatment to be targeted to the patient. Time constraints and heterogeneity of presentation complicate this process. Based on earlier consensus statements, a standardized classification scheme has been promulgated by the International

Dr. Friedman is supported through a career development award (1K23NS051409) from the National Institute of Neurological Disorders and Stroke.

[a] Department of Emergency Medicine, Albert Einstein College of Medicine, Montefiore Medical Center, 111 East 210th Street, Bronx, NY 10467, USA

[b] Department of Neurology, Albert Einstein College of Medicine, Montefiore Medical Center Headache Unit, 111 East 210th Street, Bronx, NY 10467, USA

* Corresponding author.

E-mail address: befriedm@montefiore.org (B.W. Friedman).

Headache Society to diagnose the underlying recurrent headache disorder; the second edition of the International Classification of Headache Disorders is now several years old.[5] These classification criteria are most applicable to a between-attack assessment of a patient's typical headache but are often applied to the acute attack.

Providing a diagnosis for every patient is easier said than done. Up to one third of patients who present to an ED with headache cannot be assigned a specific diagnosis, despite a thorough questionnaire-based assessment.[3] When considering an acute headache attack in isolation, rather than as representative of an underlying headache disorder, assigning a diagnosis becomes more difficult because there is often something different about the acute headache that caused a patient to present to an ED. Given the limitations of conducting a thorough history and physical examination on a patient in the throes of an acute headache, it is less likely that a complete assessment can be obtained before treatment. Once the acute headache has been controlled, taking the time to make an accurate diagnosis may facilitate the outpatient care of the patient.

MIGRAINE

Migraine is common, underdiagnosed, and treatable.[6] It affects more than one in four women, is less frequent in men, and is a leading cause of workplace absenteeism.[7,8] Migraine has a peak incidence in the third decade of life and declines with age. It can be present at the extremes of age.[8] Patients who have fewer socioeconomic resources are more likely to be underdiagnosed and undertreated.[9] Despite widespread underdiagnosis and undertreatment, the vast majority of patients who have migraine do not use an ED over the course of a year.[10] A small subset of United States migraineurs account for all ED visits, and the minority of ED users account for the majority of ED visits because these patients make multiple visits over the course of the year.[11]

A theoretic model of ED use for migraine has been proposed: patients present to an ED with their "first or worst" headache or their "last straw" headache.[12] The severe first or worst headache is generally believed to require a thorough diagnostic evaluation in the ED.[13] The last straw syndrome refers to an unbearable or unremitting exacerbation of a chronic episodic headache disorder. There is some variability in what constitutes the last straw, however; a consistent and substantial minority of urban ED headache users present to the ED without taking any analgesic, not even acetaminophen, before presenting to the ED.[14,15] In general, ED use for headache is most closely associated with ED use for other chief complaints; thus patients who rely on the ED as a source of medical care use it for management of their headache also.[11,16] Other important predictors of ED use are lower socioeconomic status and increased severity of the underlying recurrent headache disorder.[11,16]

Patients who have migraine typically give a history of a recurring, unilateral headache manifesting in attacks lasting 4 to 72 hours if not treated. Typical attacks reach moderate or severe intensity, are throbbing, are aggravated by routine physical activity, and are associated with nausea, vomiting, photophobia, phonophobia, and olfactophobia.[5] Because the standard criteria require 10 questions to diagnose migraine, various screening instruments have been developed to help clinicians identify migraine. Migraine is the headache type with many evidence-based treatment options. Using a headache expert's clinical gestalt as the gold standard, brief instruments such as IDMigraine can help identify migraine with a high degree of sensitivity.[17] IDMigraine incorporates 3 questions (nausea, photophobia, and headache-related functional disability), requires 2 to be positive, and is focused on typical attacks, rather than the acute attack. A systematic review identified the following clinical features to be most useful for discriminating migraine from nonmigraine recurrent headaches: pounding headache, duration of headache lasting 4 to 72 hours, unilateral pain, nausea, and headache-related functional disability. The presence of any four made it highly likely that the headache was indeed a migraine; fewer than three decreased the odds of migraine.[18] These instruments have yet to be validated in the ED setting, but may provide a useful frame of reference for the emergency physician.

An ED history and physical examination should focus on excluding secondary causes of headache, then determining which therapeutic agent is most appropriate. Physicians should be vigilant not to dismiss a diagnosis of migraine because of the presence of a coexisting illness, such as sinusitis.[19,20] This condition, among others, may exacerbate an acute attack of migraine. It is well recognized that acute sinusitis can indeed cause headache, although it is less clear that chronic sinusitis does the same.[19] The role of imaging in sinus headache and how to interpret the findings is not clear because findings on CT imaging of the sinuses may not correlate with a patient's symptomatology.[21,22] Surprisingly, a sizable number of patients who are either self-diagnosed with sinus headache or referred to an otolaryngology practice with this working diagnosis actually meet criteria for migraine and respond appropriately to migraine-specific medications.[23-25]

Similarly, the pain associated with a migraine headache may cause an elevation in blood pressure. Care should be taken not to mistakenly diagnose this occurrence as a hypertensive headache. Whether and how often hypertension causes headache is uncertain—even more so at levels of hypertension that are considered moderate. We believe that known migraineurs who present with an acute migraine attack and associated moderate hypertension should be treated with an analgesic medication before an antihypertensive agent if there is no evidence of end-organ damage. Physicians should be careful not to cause an unnecessary precipitous drop in blood pressure. Once the headache has been controlled the blood pressure can be reassessed and a more thorough history obtained and examination undertaken.

Diagnostic testing is of limited value in patients who have a well-established diagnosis of migraine. Concomitant infection or associated dehydration can be diagnosed clinically. Depending on the choice of therapeutic agent, pregnancy may need to be excluded before initiating therapy. In the absence of a concerning alteration in a patient's typical chronic headache pattern, emergent neuroimaging is unlikely to be helpful.

Treatment

A wide variety of treatment options is available for acute migraine, many with FDA approval and many that are used off-label. Many emergency practitioners settle on a favorite treatment, which they rely on for most cases. The ideal migraine agent would relieve the pain and associated symptoms of migraine headache rapidly and completely, without causing severe, debilitating, or frequent side effects. It would minimize the recurrence of headache after ED discharge, the likelihood of ED recidivism, and the risk for development of chronic headache. With these therapeutic goals in mind, we review the available classes of medication commonly used to treat acute migraine.

Routine intravenous fluids may be of benefit to patients who have acute migraine, although this has not been well established. For patients who have persistent gastrointestinal symptoms intravenous rehydration is unlikely to be harmful. In general, parenteral treatment is preferred because gastric stasis and delayed absorption of medication occur during an acute migraine attack.[26]

Triptans

Despite 20 years of clinical experience with the serotonin 1B/1D receptor agonists, this class of medication still has not enjoyed widespread use in the ED setting.[27]

One explanation for this is the lack of parenteral options—to this day, sumatriptan remains the only injectable triptan available in the United States. Another likely cause of infrequent use is the perception of cardiovascular risk. Although cardiac events have been infrequent, the difficulty of risk stratifying migraine patients in acute pain may cause practitioners to choose alternates.[28] Side effects, which are often short-lived, occurred in 50% of patients receiving subcutaneous sumatriptan in the ED setting. This rate is twice that of placebo-treated patients.[29] Cheaper alternatives are available; sumatriptan will soon be available as a generic medication. Nevertheless, when it is effective, subcutaneous sumatriptan can rapidly and completely relieve migraine headache, allowing patients to return promptly to their usual daily activities.

Data from a meta-analysis demonstrate that subcutaneous sumatriptan was almost three times as likely to relieve headache as placebo.[30] By 2 hours, 60% of subjects who had sumatriptan were pain-free, versus 12% of subjects who had placebo. Sustained headache response (attaining headache relief and maintaining it for 24 hours) was achieved in 49% of sumatriptan subjects, almost three times as many as placebo. In the ED setting, the median time to headache relief with subcutaneous sumatriptan was 34 minutes.[29] A large proportion of those who respond to sumatriptan suffer a headache recurrence within 24 hours of ED discharge, however.[29]

When choosing a suitable population for subcutaneous sumatriptan, the most reasonable candidates include those who report previous response to sumatriptan. Recent literature describes a phenomenon referred to as cutaneous allodynia, which may be associated with migraine headaches.[31] Cutaneous allodynia is defined as the sensation of pain in response to normally non-noxious touch stimuli, such as brushing one's hair, taking a hot shower, or putting one's hair in a ponytail. This phenomenon, hypothetically, is a manifestation of involvement of ascending pain pathways within the central nervous system.[32] The presence of cutaneous allodynia has been associated with decreased responsiveness to subcutaneous sumatriptan.[33] This phenomenon has not been well studied outside of headache subspecialty populations and may be confounded by chronicity of the underlying headache disorder. Inadvertent administration of sumatriptan during pregnancy has not resulted in a marked increase in birth defects, although safety cannot yet be assured.[34] In pregnant patients, therefore, alternate therapies should be used. Triptan nasal sprays are available but do not yet have a well-defined role in the ED.

In summary, subcutaneous sumatriptan may be considered for the treatment of acute migraine, dosed as a one-time 6-mg dose. Additional doses are unlikely to be more effective.[35] For patients who have a history of good response to triptans, subcutaneous sumatriptan should be considered a first-line therapy. For patients who are triptan naïve, the ED setting may not be the most appropriate location for a first dose.

Dihydroergotamine

Ergotamine has been used for the treatment of migraine for more than 100 years. Its hydrogenated derivative, dihydroergotamine (DHE), has been available for more than 50 years as a parenteral option and is better tolerated than its precursor.[36] Although largely replaced by the triptans because of the latter's greater selectivity for serotonin receptors, DHE may still play a useful second-line role for some ED patients. When compared head-to-head, sumatriptan has greater initial efficacy, although DHE is less likely to allow recurrence of headache, so it may be useful in patients who have a history of recurrence after treatment.[37] DHE is often administered with an antiemetic, because it commonly induces nausea. When choosing an antiemetic, one of the antimigraine antiemetics, discussed later, is preferred.

DHE, when administered as monotherapy, is less likely than sumatriptan to relieve the pain or the functional disability associated with an acute migraine attack.[38] Both medications are associated with an assortment of adverse events, including chest pain (more common with sumatriptan), nausea (more common with DHE), drowsiness, flushing, neck stiffness, vertigo, weakness, and injection site reactions.[38] When compared with chlorpromazine, DHE alone was more likely to result in use of rescue medication.[38]

DHE can be administered in doses of 0.5 to 1 mg, infused as a slow intravenous drip. It is commonly coadministered with intravenous metoclopramide 10 mg. It should be avoided in patients who have uncontrolled hypertension, risk for atherosclerotic vascular disease, and pregnancy.

The antiemetic dopamine antagonists

An increasing evidence base demonstrates that this diverse class of medications is the most appropriate first-line treatment of acute migraine in the ED setting, although mechanistic data for this class's efficacy are still lacking. Antimigraine action is probably mediated through dopamine receptor blockade, albeit this has not yet been demonstrated.

Antimigraine efficacy has been well demonstrated in multiple high-quality clinical trials for chlorpromazine,[39] metoclopramide,[14,40] prochlorperazine,[41] and droperidol.[42] In general, these medications are inexpensive, well tolerated, and at least as efficacious, if not more so, than any agent to which they have been compared. These medications should therefore be considered first-line therapy for acute migraine in the ED setting.

Of the four agents mentioned above, chlorpromazine has fallen out of favor because of profound orthostasis that may accompany administration of this medication. Of the remaining three agents, droperidol is probably the most effective, with 2-hour headache relief rates approaching 100%. The ideal dose, as determined by a high-quality dose-finding study, is 2.5 mg.[42] This medication is commonly used and exceedingly safe, but a recent FDA warning about QT prolongation has caused some clinicians to perform an EKG before medication administration.

Prochlorperazine administered in doses of 10 mg is also highly effective, although not quite as effective as droperidol.[43,44] Metoclopramide is typically administered as a 10-mg intravenous dose but has been well tolerated and efficacious when administered as repeated successive doses of 20 mg.[14,45]

Metoclopramide, prochlorperazine, and droperidol can all be accompanied by extrapyramidal symptoms, particularly akathisia, which often goes unrecognized. Prophylactic administration of diphenhydramine is a reasonable course of action, as are slower intravenous drip rates.[46,47]

The antiemetic trimethobenzamide[48] and the antipsychotic haloperidol[49] have also demonstrated efficacy and tolerability for acute migraine attacks, although as of this writing, fewer data are available to determine the relative efficacy of these two agents.

Metoclopramide has a favorable pregnancy rating and a long history of use for treatment of hyperemesis gravidarum. It is the most appropriate parenteral agent for treatment of acute migraine in pregnancy.

Nonsteroidal anti-inflammatory drugs

Nonsteroidal anti-inflammatory drugs are a mainstay of outpatient migraine therapy, particularly for less severe migraine attacks. The parenteral nonsteroidal ketorolac has demonstrated efficacy for the acute treatment of migraine. Its overall efficacy is comparable to meperidine,[50–52] although less than the antiemetics.[53–55] In patients who do not have contraindications to nonsteroidals, such as peptic ulcer disease or chronic kidney disease, this medication dosed at 30 mg intravenously or 60 mg intramuscularly is a reasonable treatment option, either as primary treatment or as adjuvant therapy for acute migraine.

Opioids

Opioids, particularly meperidine, are still the most widely used medications for the treatment of acute migraine in North American EDs.[27,56] Standard critiques of opioid use for migraine include the following: decreased efficacy, high rate of adverse effects, increased rate of recurrence of migraine within the short term, increased rate of ED recidivism, and association with chronic migraine, although specific data for all of these are underwhelming. A recent meta-analysis demonstrated that meperidine is less efficacious for the treatment of acute migraine and burdened by more side effects than regimens containing DHE.[57] Additionally, meperidine is probably less efficacious than the antiemetics; it allows a higher rate of return visits to the ED but a lower rate of extrapyramidal side effects. Meperidine is no better than ketorolac, with a similar side-effect profile.[57] Some data suggest that meperidine is associated with an increased rate of return visit to the ED[56,58] and may be associated with decreased responsiveness to triptans.[59] In short, there are ample reasons to recommend avoidance of meperidine as a first-line treatment of migraine. In patients who have infrequent episodic migraine and a history of excellent response to this medication, it still may be a reasonable option.

When choosing among opioids, scant data are available to help guide a clinician. Parenteral morphine and hydromorphone have not been subjected to comparative clinical trials. Intramuscular butorphanol is more efficacious than meperidine and is as efficacious and well tolerated as DHE plus metoclopramide.[60] Opioids should not be withheld on principle; in general, this class of medication is highly effective, safe, and well tolerated for the management of acute pain. For this one ailment, however, better agents are available.

Valproic acid

A more recent addition to the antimigraine armamentarium, this antiepileptic medication has seemed beneficial in open-label studies,[61–63] although it has performed less well in randomized trials.[64] It is not an unreasonable choice as a final treatment before admission but should not be considered a first-line medication. Valproic acid is often administered in doses between 500 mg and 1 g as a slow intravenous drip over 30 minutes.

Recurrence of Migraine After Emergency Department Discharge

No matter the treatment used, migraines frequently recur after ED discharge. Two thirds of patients report headache within 24 hours of ED discharge; half of these are moderate or severe in intensity. Fifty percent of patients report functional disability within 24 hours of ED discharge.[65,66] It is difficult to predict who will suffer headache after discharge. Risk factors include a history of headache recurrence, longer duration of headache, more severe pain at baseline, or persistent pain at discharge. It is reasonable to educate all patients as to the likelihood of recurrence.

A recent meta-analysis demonstrated that one dose of parenteral dexamethasone administered in the ED can decrease the rate of recurrence of headache after ED discharge, with a number needed to treat of nine.[67] Dexamethasone may begin to be effective within several hours. Doses of dexamethasone demonstrating efficacy have ranged from 10 to 24 mg, without a clear dose-response curve. In general, one dose of dexamethasone was well tolerated, and may now be considered first-line therapy to decrease the recurrence of headache after ED discharge.

It is less clear what additional medications should be offered to treat the recurrence of headache after ED discharge. Nonsteroidals, such as naproxen, or triptans, such as sumatriptan, are reasonable options, although data are not available.

A substantial proportion of migraine patients who use the ED continue to suffer from their underlying headache disorder over the months after ED discharge.[66] It is reasonable practice to start patients who suffer from episodic migraines on an oral medication for use during their next migraine attack, particularly if neurology or headache specialty appointments are difficult to obtain. If nonsteroidals, acetaminophen, or aspirin have not proved sufficient for the patient previously, consider starting the patient on a triptan medication, assuming low cardiovascular risk, or a combination of metoclopramide taken with a nonsteroidal drug or salicylate. An evidence-based approach to outpatient care stratifies patients based on headache-related disability at baseline.[68] Patients who have substantial headache-related functional disability at baseline (ie, frequently miss work or social activities) benefit from a triptan and patients who do not have as much functional disability can be started on cheaper alternatives, such as a prescription nonsteroidal with or without metoclopramide. Although baseline headache-related functional disability scores are less useful in the ED setting, this model is a useful framework to approach migraine care at the time of discharge.

Frequent Emergency Department Migraine Visitors

Although they represent fewer than 10% of all ED headache patients, frequent ED users account for 50% of visits in some institutions.[69] The reasons patients frequent the ED are not well understood. Although it could represent drug-seeking behavior, it may also be a marker for poorly treated migraine. Headache patients who frequent the ED tend to know their disease well and request specific medications, often opioids. Although effective ED-based approaches to the frequent visitor have not been reported in the headache literature, individual EDs should develop a uniform departmental approach to the chronic pain patient so that the pain and social needs of the patient can be addressed appropriately. Physician-to-physician variability in management leads to unpleasant confrontations for the physician and uncomfortable situations for the patients, who at times are forced to beg for analgesia within the throes of an acute migraine.

Some data demonstrate a decrease in the frequency of ED visits for patients who have chronic headache who participated in a comprehensive headache management program that offered headache education and multidisciplinary care.[70–72] These programs were effective at decreasing the burden of illness and health care costs in patients who had chronic headaches, though only select patients were able to benefit from these programs.

We could not find any evidence-based ED-appropriate strategies for addressing a patient's opioid for migraine requirements from the perspective of the individual clinician. This problem is difficult for an emergency clinician in the middle of a busy shift. Potential strategies include offering a nonopioid therapy in conjunction with a lower opioid dose, referring to an appropriate outpatient clinician, and initiating a preventative therapy at the time of discharge. It is not clear how best to handle infrequent ED users who report complete and persistent relief after one dose of opioid. One should not deny effective analgesics to patients who respond well to a particular therapy, but there is an association between this particular class of therapy, chronic migraine, and ED recidivism.

Special Concerns for a Pediatric Population

Migraine incidence begins to peak in early adolescence[6] and may be a concern for children as young as 5 or 6 years of age. In general, the presentation of pediatric migraine is more atypical; children may present with bilateral headache of shorter duration and without the combination of photo- and phonophobia.[73] There is a smaller evidence base for the treatment of pediatric migraine, partly because of a high placebo-response rate in this population. Management of pediatric migraine often consists of simple analgesics, such as ibuprofen or acetaminophen, which seem to be as efficacious in this population as oral triptans.[74,75] The antiemetic dopamine antagonists are commonly used,[76] although efficacy data are inferential and limited to prochlorperazine.[53] The pediatric population also suffers several variants of cyclical pediatric pain and vomiting syndromes linked to migraine. These are particularly difficult to diagnose because they lack associated headache. Cyclical vomiting, benign paroxysmal vertigo of childhood, and abdominal migraine are associated with development of migraine in adulthood.[5]

TENSION-TYPE HEADACHE

Although common in the general population, tension-type headache is rarely severe and only infrequently causes an ED visit.[77] This headache is defined by the absence of migraine's characteristic features, such as nausea, vomiting, severe intensity, or causing functional disability.[5] The pain is typically bilateral, pressing or tightening in quality, and of mild to moderate intensity. Generally, the pain does not worsen with routine physical activity. There is some controversy as to whether this headache is indeed a distinct illness or merely a milder form of migraine. Speaking against this shared pathophysiology argument are distinct epidemiologic data; in contrast to migraine, tension-type headache is a disease of higher socioeconomic demographics.[8,77] Speaking for a unified pathophysiology is a shared response to many of the same medications that are effective against migraine, such as triptans, antiemetics, and nonsteroidals.[78–80]

Traditional management of tension-type headache calls for nonsteroidals, which have a solid background of efficacy in this illness. Limited but methodologically sound data demonstrate efficacy of chlorpromazine and metoclopramide for the treatment of tension-type headache also.[78,81] Sumatriptan has also demonstrated efficacy in ED patients who have tension-type headache and in outpatients who have severe episodic tension-type headache if they have an underlying migraine disorder.[79,80] In general, once the emergency physician has excluded secondary headache from the differential diagnosis, it would be appropriate to treat the acute headache with an antiemetic, such as metoclopramide.

Like migraine, tension-type headache remains a problem after ED discharge. Nineteen percent of patients who have tension-type headache treated in an ED reported moderate or severe headache within 24 hours of discharge; 23% report headache-related functional impairment.[66] The emergency physician should ensure that the initial headache is well treated and that the patient has adequate resources to treat the recurrence of headache after ED discharge.

CLUSTER

Cluster is a rare headache[82] and an infrequent cause of ED presentation, particularly when compared with migraine or tension-type headache. An accurate diagnosis allows for effective treatment and helps avoid unnecessary diagnostic and therapeutic interventions. Barriers to accurate diagnosis include the brevity of the attacks, which may have ended before ED evaluation, the rarity of the disorder and consequent lack of physician familiarity with its presentation, and the lack of specificity of the autonomic features, which may cause physicians to think of other illnesses.[83]

Classically a disease of men,[83] this illness usually begins between the ages of 20 and 40 years.[84] The most common type is episodic cluster, in which headaches occur in groups or clusters lasting weeks to months and are followed by headache-free periods or remissions lasting one month or longer. Approximately 10% of patients who have cluster headache either do not experience remissions or have remissions lasting less than 1 month. In these cases, the term "chronic cluster headache" is applied.

The pain of cluster headache is invariably unilateral and the side affected generally is consistent for every attack and every cluster period (the interval of time containing sequential attacks). Predominantly situated in and around the eye and temporal locations, the pain may radiate into the ipsilateral neck, ear, cheek, jaw, upper and lower teeth, and nose.[85] The latter areas, if involved, may account for unnecessary dental and sinus investigations and treatments.

The pain is excruciating in intensity and is typically described as a stabbing or boring sensation, similar to a hot poker being thrust into the eye. An attack begins abruptly and rapidly intensifies, reaching a climax of pain within 5 to 15 minutes. The attack also ceases suddenly and the patient often is left feeling exhausted. The presence of at least one accompanying cranial autonomic symptom is a criterion for the diagnosis of cluster headache.[5] Autonomic features include conjunctival injection, lacrimation, nasal congestion, rhinorrhea, eyelid edema, forehead and facial sweating, ptosis, and miosis. These signs are invariably ipsilateral to the side of the pain.

Another notable feature of cluster headache is its short duration. Each untreated attack typically lasts from 15 to 180 minutes, with more than 75% of attacks reported lasting less than 60 minutes. Because of the brevity of each attack, a partial or complete recovery may have occurred by the time of evaluation in the ED; this can obscure the correct diagnosis. Attacks rarely may last longer than 3 hours. Attacks commonly occur one to three times daily, although they may be as variable as one every other day to up to eight daily. The daily attacks usually last for 2 to 3 months (the cluster period). The headaches then remit spontaneously, only to recur again as another cluster of daily headaches months to years later.[86]

There is usually a remarkable predictability to the timing of the individual attack and the cluster period, a phenomenon that distinguishes cluster headache from other primary headache disorders. Specific questioning often reveals its circadian and circannual periodicity, when daily attacks recur at the same time each day and cluster periods occur at the same time each year. Furthermore, there is a predilection for headaches to occur at night; the attacks often awaken the sufferer 90 minutes after falling asleep, corresponding to the onset of the first period of rapid eye movement (REM) sleep. Sleep deprivation often is a result of these repeated nightly attacks and may trigger additional attacks. Alcoholic beverages and vasodilator medications, such as nitroglycerin, also may trigger an attack during the cluster period.[84] Seasonal periodicity is observed frequently, with the highest incidence of cluster periods occurring in the spring and autumn.

In contrast to migraineurs, sufferers of cluster headache are agitated and restless and prefer to be erect and to move about; sufferers of migraine prefer to lie quietly in a dark room. The intensity of the pain may cause some patients to wail loudly and others may engage in destructive activities, such as banging their heads against the wall. The pain is so excruciating that it may drive cluster headache sufferers to suicide.[86]

ED-based treatment should be directed at relieving the acute attack and aborting the entire cluster of headaches. Abortive agents for cluster headache must work quickly and effectively. For most patients suffering from an acute cluster attack, the use of oxygen inhalation is the treatment of choice because it is easily administered, has an excellent safety profile, and works rapidly.[87,88] In our experience, oxygen is most effective when administered with the patient bent forward in a seated position through a loose-fitting, non-rebreathing facial mask at a flow rate of 7 to 10 L/min for 15 minutes. The response usually is rapid and appreciable, benefiting roughly 70% of patients within 15 minutes. Although it is unclear why flow rate should matter when breathing 100% oxygen from a non-rebreather device, increasing the flow rate of oxygen to 15 L/min has been reported to help those refractory to the initial intervention.[89] Administering oxygen at the pinnacle of the attack may reduce the pain significantly; delivering it close to the onset of the attack may abort the pain completely. Subcutaneous sumatriptan in doses up to 12 mg subcutaneously is highly effective at relieving cluster headache, although because of increased adverse effects, 6 mg is a more appropriate dose.[90] Subcutaneous sumatriptan has a rapid onset and is considered to be the most effective abortive agent for acute cluster attacks, often producing a benefit in 5 to 7 minutes after administration. A 6-mg subcutaneous dose may be repeated at least 1 hour later but not more than twice daily. DHE at doses of 0.5 to 1.0 mg given intravenously or intramuscularly is also useful as an abortive agent for cluster headache, although evidence supporting this medication is lacking. Antiemetic dopamine receptor antagonists may be useful for acute attacks.[91,92] Subcutaneous octreotide (somatostatin) dosed at 100 µg can abort the acute attack, with a number needed to treat of five for complete relief of headache by 30 minutes.[93]

After successful management of the individual episode of cluster headache, patients should be given treatment recommendations and referred to a qualified specialist. Because cluster headache is a condition of relatively long duration, follow-up care and prophylaxis are essential to avoid repeat visits to the ED for each attack of cluster. The patient should be reassured that there is no underlying organic pathology responsible for their headache.

Avoidance of potential triggers of cluster headache is recommended. During the active cluster period, patients should be advised to refrain from taking daytime naps, drinking alcoholic beverages, and using medications, such as nitroglycerin, that are vasodilators and can trigger attacks. Recurrence of symptoms is common within 24 hours of the ED visit; therefore, consideration should be given to starting the patient on transitional and maintenance therapy. Prescriptions may also be written for subcutaneous sumatriptan, oxygen, or both so that the patient is able to treat acute attacks at home. Corticosteroids are often recommended as transitional treatment of cluster headache, although the evidence base for this treatment is underwhelming.[94,95] Verapamil has been shown to be an effective prophylactic agent for cluster headache.[96] If rapid follow-up with a headache specialist cannot be ensured, these medications should be initiated in the ED.

OTHER PRIMARY HEADACHES

Less common, and more difficult to diagnosis, are various benign recurrent headache disorders whose initial presentation can be concerning. Secondary mimics of these disorders must be excluded.

Primary Cough Headache

This headache is brought on suddenly by coughing, straining, or other Valsalva maneuvers.[5] The pain has been described as sharp, stabbing, or splitting in nature, moderate to severe in intensity, and maximal in the vertex, frontal, occipital, or temporal regions. The headache lasts from 1 second to 30 minutes. Approximately one half of all cases of cough headache are attributable to secondary causes. Diagnostic neuroimaging, with special attention to the posterior fossa and base of the skull, is therefore mandatory to differentiate secondary and primary forms of cough headache. Indomethacin may help patients who frequently experience cough headache.[97]

Primary Exertional Headache

This headache begins shortly after exertion.[5] In one ED case series, four cases were identified over a 6-month period, all in men, and all provoked by lifting weights.[98] Headache typically last up to 1 day. Treatment is avoidance of the instigating activity, although nonsteroidals taken before exertion may be of benefit.

Postcoital Headache or Headache Associated with Sexual Activity

Usually this headache is described as severe and explosive. Because of this presentation, other types of headache with a potential for malignant course need to be excluded.[5] Headache provoked by sexual activity usually begins as a dull bilateral ache as sexual excitement increases, and suddenly becomes intense at orgasm. Two subtypes are classified: pre-orgasmic headache, a dull ache in the head and neck, and orgasmic headache, an explosive and severe headache occurring with orgasm.[99] The mainstay of treatment of this headache disorder is usually reassurance, although preemptive treatment with indomethacin or prophylaxis with a beta-blocker may prevent attacks.

Primary Thunderclap Headache

This disorder is characterized by a severe headache that begins abruptly and rapidly intensifies, reaching a climax of pain within 1 minute.[100] The pain is most commonly occipital in location, but may involve any region of the head and neck. Associated symptoms may include migrainous features. The pain lasts from 1 hour to 10 days and may recur within the first week after onset but not regularly over subsequent weeks or months. This diagnosis can be established only after excluding secondary headache disorders.

HEMICRANIA CONTINUA

Hemicrania continua is characterized as a continuous, strictly unilateral headache of mild to moderate intensity with superimposed exacerbations of more severe pain. During these exacerbations, one or more autonomic symptoms (ptosis, conjunctival injection, lacrimation, and nasal congestion) occur ipsilateral to the pain. Many patients report a foreign body sensation, like an eyelash or a piece of sand, in the eye ipsilateral to the pain. This headache is defined by its absolute response to therapeutic doses of indomethacin.

NEW DAILY PERSISTENT HEADACHE

This disorder is characterized by a daily and unremitting headache that becomes continuous shortly (<3 days) after onset, without a precipitating factor or a prior headache history. A clear recall of such an onset is necessary to establish the diagnosis of daily persistent headache (NDPH). It has features of both migraine and tension-type headache. It seems that there may be subtypes of NDPH: a self-limited form, which typically resolves spontaneously without treatment, and a refractory form, which is associated with an inconsistent and suboptimal response regardless of the therapeutic modality used. Two of the most common identifiable secondary causes of NDPH are spontaneous cerebrospinal fluid leaks and cerebral venous sinus thrombosis.

MEDICATION OVERUSE HEADACHE

Frequent analgesic use is now well recognized as an independent cause of chronic daily headache.[5] The cycle begins when over-the-counter or prescription medication is used with increasing frequency to treat a primary headache disorder, ultimately causing a dependence on the medication and a lack of response to acute therapies that formerly were effective. This syndrome has been reported with a wide variety of anti-headache medications, including acetaminophen, ergotamine, opioids, and triptans.[101] Although these patients may have to be admitted for detoxification, an outpatient regimen consisting of a novel acute therapy and a migraine preventative may be appropriate. This headache is difficult to diagnose and requires a detailed assessment of the patient's headache history and medication use. It has a high relapse rate; if outpatient therapy is considered, the care should be coordinated with the outpatient physician.

WHEN TO CONSIDER ADMISSION: THE INTRACTABLE HEADACHE

Despite aggressive ED management, some headaches do not remit, or they return rapidly after initial therapy. Admission to an inpatient unit for comprehensive headache management and control of external stressors may be needed to abort the headache successfully. Various inpatient regimens are used, all of which incorporate classes of medication discussed above. The Raskin protocol, consisting of around-the-clock administration of parenteral antiemetics and DHE, has been used successfully for almost 2 decades.[102]

REFERENCES

1. Goldstein JN, Camargo CA Jr, Pelletier AJ, et al. Headache in United States emergency departments: demographics, work-up and frequency of pathological diagnoses. Cephalalgia 2006;26(6):684–90.
2. Bigal M, Bordini CA, Speciali JG. Headache in an emergency room in Brazil. Sao Paulo Med J 2000;118(3):58–62.
3. Friedman BW, Hochberg ML, Esses D, et al. Applying the International Classification of Headache Disorders to the emergency department: an assessment of reproducibility and the frequency with which a unique diagnosis can be assigned to every acute headache presentation. Ann Emerg Med 2007;49(4): 409–19.
4. Luda E, Comitangelo R, Sicuro L. The symptom of headache in emergency departments. The experience of a neurology emergency department. Ital J Neurol Sci 1995;16(5):295–301.
5. The Classification Subcommittee of the International Headache Society. The international classification of headache disorders. 2nd edition. Cephalalgia 2004; 24(Suppl 1):1–160.
6. Lipton RB, Diamond S, Reed M, et al. Migraine diagnosis and treatment: results from the American Migraine Study II. Headache 2001;41(7):638–45.
7. Hu XH, Markson LE, Lipton RB, et al. Burden of migraine in the United States: disability and economic costs. Arch Intern Med 1999;159(8):813–8.

8. Lipton RB, Scher AI, Kolodner K, et al. Migraine in the United States: epidemiology and patterns of health care use. Neurology 2002;58(6): 885–94.
9. Lipton RB, Stewart WF, Diamond S, et al. Prevalence and burden of migraine in the United States: data from the American Migraine Study II. Headache 2001; 41(7):646–57.
10. Celentano DD, Stewart WF, Lipton RB, et al. Medication use and disability among migraineurs: a national probability sample survey. Headache 1992; 32(5):223–8.
11. Friedman BW, Reed ML, Serrano D, et al. Frequency of emergency department or urgent care use: results from the American Migraine Prevalence and Prevention study (abstract). Headache 2007;47(5):745–6.
12. Edmeads J. Emergency management of headache. Headache 1988;28(10):675–9.
13. Edlow JA, Caplan LR. Avoiding pitfalls in the diagnosis of subarachnoid hemorrhage. N Engl J Med 2000;342(1):29–36.
14. Friedman BW, Corbo J, Lipton RB, et al. A trial of metoclopramide vs sumatriptan for the emergency department treatment of migraines. Neurology 2005; 64(3):463–8.
15. Salomone JA 3rd, Thomas RW, Althoff JR, et al. An evaluation of the role of the ED in the management of migraine headaches. Am J Emerg Med 1994;12(2): 134–7.
16. Lane PL, Nituica CM, Sorondo B. Headache patients: who does not come to the emergency department? (abstract). Acad Emerg Med 2003;10(5): 528.
17. Lipton RB, Dodick D, Sadovsky R, et al. A self-administered screener for migraine in primary care: The ID Migraine™ validation study. Neurology 2003; 61(3):375–82.
18. Detsky ME, McDonald DR, Baerlocher MO, et al. Does this patient with headache have a migraine or need neuroimaging? JAMA 2006;296(10):1274–83.
19. Cady RK, Dodick DW, Levine HL, et al. Sinus headache: a neurology, otolaryngology, allergy, and primary care consensus on diagnosis and treatment. Mayo Clin Proc 2005;80(7):908–16.
20. Cady RK, Schreiber CP. Sinus headache or migraine? Considerations in making a differential diagnosis. Neurology 2002;58(9 Suppl 6):S10–4.
21. Bhattacharyya T, Piccirillo J, Wippold FJ 2nd. Relationship between patient-based descriptions of sinusitis and paranasal sinus computed tomographic findings. Arch Otolaryngol Head Neck Surg 1997;123(11):1189–92.
22. Shields G, Seikaly H, LeBoeuf M, et al. Correlation between facial pain or headache and computed tomography in rhinosinusitis in Canadian and U.S. subjects. Laryngoscope 2003;113(6):943–5.
23. Eross E, Dodick D, Eross M. The Sinus, Allergy and Migraine Study (SAMS). Headache 2007;47(2):213–24.
24. Ishkanian G, Blumenthal H, Webster CJ, et al. Efficacy of sumatriptan tablets in migraineurs self-described or physician-diagnosed as having sinus headache: a randomized, double-blind, placebo-controlled study. Clin Ther 2007;29(1): 99–109.
25. Schreiber CP, Hutchinson S, Webster CJ, et al. Prevalence of migraine in patients with a history of self-reported or physician-diagnosed "sinus" headache. Arch Intern Med 2004;164(16):1769–72.
26. Aurora S, Kori S, Barrodale P, et al. Gastric stasis occurs in spontaneous, visually induced, and interictal migraine. Headache 2007;47(10):1443–6.

27. Vinson DR. Treatment patterns of isolated benign headache in US emergency departments. Ann Emerg Med 2002;39(3):215–22.

28. Dodick D, Lipton RB, Martin V, et al. Consensus statement: cardiovascular safety profile of triptans (5-HT agonists) in the acute treatment of migraine. Headache 2004;44(5):414–25.

29. Akpunonu BE, Mutgi AB, Federman DJ, et al. Subcutaneous sumatriptan for treatment of acute migraine in patients admitted to the emergency department: a multicenter study. Ann Emerg Med 1995;25(4):464–9.

30. Oldman AD, Smith LA, McQuay HJ, et al. Pharmacological treatments for acute migraine: quantitative systematic review. Pain 2002;97(3):247–57.

31. Burstein R, Yarnitsky D, Goor-Aryeh I, et al. An association between migraine and cutaneous allodynia. Ann Neurol 2000;47(5):614–24.

32. Dodick D, Silberstein S. Central sensitization theory of migraine: clinical implications. Headache 2006;46(Suppl 4):S182–91.

33. Burstein R, Collins B, Jakubowski M. Defeating migraine pain with triptans: a race against the development of cutaneous allodynia. Ann Neurol 2004;55(1):19–26.

34. Loder E. Safety of sumatriptan in pregnancy: a review of the data so far. CNS Drugs 2003;17(1):1–7.

35. Treatment of migraine attacks with sumatriptan. The Subcutaneous Sumatriptan International Study Group. N Engl J Med 1991;325(5):316–21.

36. Silberstein SD, McCrory DC. Ergotamine and dihydroergotamine: history, pharmacology, and efficacy. Headache 2003;43(2):144–66.

37. Winner P, Ricalde O, Le Force B, et al. A double-blind study of subcutaneous dihydroergotamine vs subcutaneous sumatriptan in the treatment of acute migraine. Arch Neurol 1996;53(2):180–4.

38. Colman I, Brown MD, Innes GD, et al. Parenteral dihydroergotamine for acute migraine headache: a systematic review of the literature. Ann Emerg Med 2005;45(4):393–401.

39. Bigal ME, Bordini CA, Speciali JG. Intravenous chlorpromazine in the emergency department treatment of migraines: a randomized controlled trial. J Emerg Med 2002;23(2):141–8.

40. Colman I, Brown MD, Innes GD, et al. Parenteral metoclopramide for acute migraine: meta-analysis of randomised controlled trials. BMJ 2004;329(7479):1369–73.

41. Jones J, Sklar D, Dougherty J, et al. Randomized double-blind trial of intravenous prochlorperazine for the treatment of acute headache. JAMA 1989; 261(8):1174–6.

42. Silberstein SD, Young WB, Mendizabal JE, et al. Acute migraine treatment with droperidol: a randomized, double-blind, placebo-controlled trial. Neurology 2003;60(2):315–21.

43. Miner JR, Fish SJ, Smith SW, et al. Droperidol vs. prochlorperazine for benign headaches in the emergency department. Acad Emerg Med 2001;8(9):873–9.

44. Weaver CS, Jones JB, Chisholm CD, et al. Droperidol vs prochlorperazine for the treatment of acute headache. J Emerg Med 2004;26(2):145–50.

45. Corbo J, Esses D, Bijur PE, et al. Randomized clinical trial of intravenous magnesium sulfate as an adjunctive medication for emergency department treatment of migraine headache. Ann Emerg Med 2001;38(6):621–7.

46. Vinson DR. Diphenhydramine in the treatment of akathisia induced by prochlorperazine. J Emerg Med 2004;26(3):265–70.

47. Vinson DR, Migala AF, Quesenberry CP Jr. Slow infusion for the prevention of akathisia induced by prochlorperazine: a randomized controlled trial. J Emerg Med 2001;20(2):113–9.

48. Friedman BW, Hochberg M, Esses D, et al. A clinical trial of trimethobenzamide/diphenhydramine versus sumatriptan for acute migraines. Headache 2006; 46(6):934–41.
49. Honkaniemi J, Liimatainen S, Rainesalo S, et al. Haloperidol in the acute treatment of migraine: a randomized, double-blind, placebo-controlled study. Headache 2006;46(5):781–7.
50. Davis CP, Torre PR, Williams C, et al. Ketorolac versus meperidine-plus-promethazine treatment of migraine headache: evaluations by patients. Am J Emerg Med 1995;13(2):146–50.
51. Duarte C, Dunaway F, Turner L, et al. Ketorolac versus meperidine and hydroxyzine in the treatment of acute migraine headache: a randomized, prospective, double-blind trial. Ann Emerg Med 1992;21(9):1116–21.
52. Larkin GL, Prescott JE. A randomized, double-blind, comparative study of the efficacy of ketorolac tromethamine versus meperidine in the treatment of severe migraine. Ann Emerg Med 1992;21(8):919–24.
53. Brousseau DC, Duffy SJ, Anderson AC, et al. Treatment of pediatric migraine headaches: a randomized, double-blind trial of prochlorperazine versus ketorolac. Ann Emerg Med 2004;43(2):256–62.
54. Klapper JA, Stanton JS. Ketorolac versus DHE and metoclopramide in the treatment of migraine headaches. Headache 1991;31(8):523–4.
55. Seim MB, March JA, Dunn KA. Intravenous ketorolac vs intravenous prochlorperazine for the treatment of migraine headaches. Acad Emerg Med 1998; 5(6):573–6.
56. Colman I, Rothney A, Wright SC, et al. Use of narcotic analgesics in the emergency department treatment of migraine headache. Neurology 2004;62(10):1695–700.
57. Friedman BW, Friedman MS, Hochberg ML, et al. The relative efficacy of meperidine for acute migraine. A meta-analysis (abstract). Acad Emerg Med 2008; 15(5).
58. Stiell IG, Dufour DG, Moher D, et al. Methotrimeprazine versus meperidine and dimenhydrinate in the treatment of severe migraine: a randomized, controlled trial. Ann Emerg Med 1991;20(11):1201–5.
59. Jakubowski M, Levy D, Goor-Aryeh I, et al. Terminating migraine with allodynia and ongoing central sensitization using parenteral administration of COX1/COX2 inhibitors. Headache 2005;45(7):850–61.
60. Belgrade MJ, Ling LJ, Schleevogt MB, et al. Comparison of single-dose meperidine, butorphanol, and dihydroergotamine in the treatment of vascular headache. Neurology 1989;39(4):590–2.
61. Edwards KR, Norton J, Behnke M. Comparison of intravenous valproate versus intramuscular dihydroergotamine and metoclopramide for acute treatment of migraine headache. Headache 2001;41(10):976–80.
62. Mathew NT, Kailasam J, Meadors L, et al. Intravenous valproate sodium (Depacon) aborts migraine rapidly: a preliminary report. Headache 2000;40(9):720–3.
63. Schwartz TH, Karpitskiy VV, Sohn RS. Intravenous valproate sodium in the treatment of daily headache. Headache 2002;42(6):519–22.
64. Tanen DA, Miller S, French T, et al. Intravenous sodium valproate versus prochlorperazine for the emergency department treatment of acute migraine headaches: a prospective, randomized, double-blind trial. Ann Emerg Med 2003; 41(6):847–53.
65. Ducharme J, Beveridge RC, Lee JS, et al. Emergency management of migraine: is the headache really over? Acad Emerg Med 1998;5(9):899–905.

66. Friedman B, Hochberg M, Esses D, et al. Pain and functional outcomes of patients with primary headache disorder discharged from the emergency department (abstract). Acad Emerg Med 2006;13(5 Suppl 1):S18.

67. Colman I, Friedman BW, Brown MD, et al. Parenteral dexamethasone for preventing recurrent migraine headaches: a systematic review of the literature. BMJ 2008; 336(7657):1359–61.

68. Lipton RB, Stewart WF, Stone AM, et al. Stratified care vs step care strategies for migraine: the Disability in Strategies of Care (DISC) Study: a randomized trial. JAMA 2000;284(20):2599–605.

69. Maizels M. Health resource utilization of the emergency department headache "repeater." Headache 2002;42(8):747–53.

70. Blumenfeld A, Tischio M. Center of excellence for headache care: group model at Kaiser Permanente. Headache 2003;43(5):431–40.

71. Harpole LH, Samsa GP, Jurgelski AE, et al. Headache management program improves outcome for chronic headache. Headache 2003;43(7):715–24.

72. Maizels M, Saenz V, Wirjo J. Impact of a group-based model of disease management for headache. Headache 2003;43(6):621–7.

73. Hershey AD, Winner P, Kabbouche MA, et al. Use of the ICHD-II criteria in the diagnosis of pediatric migraine. Headache 2005;45(10):1288–97.

74. Damen L, Bruijn JK, Verhagen AP, et al. Symptomatic treatment of migraine in children: a systematic review of medication trials. Pediatrics 2005;116(2): e295–302.

75. Evers S, Rahmann A, Kraemer C, et al. Treatment of childhood migraine attacks with oral zolmitriptan and ibuprofen. Neurology 2006;67(3):497–9.

76. Richer L, Graham L, Klassen T, et al. Emergency department management of acute migraine in children in Canada: a practice variation study. Headache 2007;47(5):703–10.

77. Schwartz BS, Stewart WF, Simon D, et al. Epidemiology of tension-type headache. JAMA 1998;279(5):381–3.

78. Bigal ME, Bordini CA, Speciali JG. Intravenous chlorpromazine in the acute treatment of episodic tension-type headache: a randomized, placebo controlled, double-blind study. Arq Neuropsiquiatr 2002;60(3-A):537–41.

79. Lipton RB, Stewart WF, Cady R, et al. 2000 Wolfe Award. Sumatriptan for the range of headaches in migraine sufferers: results of the spectrum study. Headache 2000;40(10):783–91.

80. Miner JR, Smith SW, Moore J, et al. Sumatriptan for the treatment of undifferentiated primary headaches in the ED. Am J Emerg Med 2007;25(1):60–4.

81. Cicek M, Karcioglu O, Parlak I, et al. Prospective, randomised, double blind, controlled comparison of metoclopramide and pethidine in the emergency treatment of acute primary vascular and tension type headache episodes. Emerg Med J 2004;21(3):323–6.

82. Sjaastad O, Bakketeig LS. Cluster headache prevalence. Vaga study of headache epidemiology. Cephalalgia 2003;23(7):528–33.

83. Bahra A, Goadsby PJ. Diagnostic delays and mis-management in cluster headache. Acta Neurol Scand 2004;109(3):175–9.

84. Manzoni GC. Cluster headache and lifestyle: remarks on a population of 374 male patients. Cephalalgia 1999;19(2):88–94.

85. Bahra A, May A, Goadsby PJ. Cluster headache: a prospective clinical study with diagnostic implications. Neurology 2002;58(3):354–61.

86. Dodick DW, Rozen TD, Goadsby PJ, et al. Cluster headache. Cephalalgia 2000; 20(9):787–803.

87. Fogan L. Treatment of cluster headache. A double-blind comparison of oxygen v air inhalation. Arch Neurol 1985;42(4):362–3.
88. Kudrow L. Response of cluster headache attacks to oxygen inhalation. Headache 1981;21(1):1–4.
89. Rozen TD. High oxygen flow rates for cluster headache. Neurology 2004;63(3): 593.
90. Treatment of acute cluster headache with sumatriptan. The Sumatriptan Cluster Headache Study Group. N Engl J Med 1991;325(5):322–6.
91. Caviness VS Jr, O'Brien P. Cluster headache: response to chlorpromazine. Headache 1980;20(3):128–31.
92. Rozen TD. Olanzapine as an abortive agent for cluster headache. Headache 2001;41(8):813–6.
93. Matharu MS, Levy MJ, Meeran K, et al. Subcutaneous octreotide in cluster headache: randomized placebo-controlled double-blind crossover study. Ann Neurol 2004;56(4):488–94.
94. Couch JR Jr, Ziegler DK. Prednisone therapy for cluster headache. Headache 1978;18(4):219–21.
95. Mir P, Alberca R, Navarro A, et al. Prophylactic treatment of episodic cluster headache with intravenous bolus of methylprednisolone. Neurol Sci 2003; 24(5):318–21.
96. Leone M, D'Amico D, Frediani F, et al. Verapamil in the prophylaxis of episodic cluster headache: a double-blind study versus placebo. Neurology 2000;54(6): 1382–5.
97. Pascual J, Iglesias F, Oterino A, et al. Cough, exertional, and sexual headaches: an analysis of 72 benign and symptomatic cases. Neurology 1996;46(6):1520–4.
98. Imperato J, Burstein J, Edlow JA. Benign exertional headache. Ann Emerg Med 2003;41(1):98–103.
99. Lance JW. Headaches related to sexual activity. J Neurol Neurosurg Psychiatry 1976;39(12):1226–30.
100. Schwedt TJ, Matharu MS, Dodick DW. Thunderclap headache. Lancet Neurol 2006;5(7):621–31.
101. Dodick D, Freitag F. Evidence-based understanding of medication-overuse headache: clinical implications. Headache 2006;46(Suppl 4):S202–11.
102. Raskin NH. Repetitive intravenous dihydroergotamine as therapy for intractable migraine. Neurology 1986;36(7):995–7.

Central Nervous System Infections

David Somand, MD[a], William Meurer, MD[a,b],*

KEYWORDS

• CNS infections • Meningitis • Encephalitis • CNS abscess

Central nervous system (CNS) infections have long been recognized as among the most devastating of diseases. Early accounts of "epidemic cerebrospinal fever" by Viesseux[1,2] in 1805 and the first American epidemic of meningococcal meningitis in 1806 were described as a nearly always fatal disease. Today, understanding of the epidemiology and pathophysiology, along with improved treatments and vaccination programs, have markedly changed the impact and outcome of the disease.[3–10]

CNS infections are varied, and definitions of disease entities are important. Meningitis is defined as inflammation of the membranes of the brain or spinal cord and is also known as arachnoiditis or leptomeningitis. Encephalitis denotes inflammation of the brain itself, whereas myelitis refers to inflammation of the spinal cord. Combinations of terms, including "meningoencephalitis" or "encephalomyelitis," refer to more diffuse processes of infection.[11] Collections of infective and purulent material may coalesce within the CNS as abscesses.

This article describes the changing pattern and epidemiology of a variety of common CNS infections, including meningitis, encephalitis, and brain abscesses, and reviews pathophysiology and the most current approach to clinical diagnosis, treatment, and disposition from the emergency physician perspective.

BACTERIAL MENINGITIS
Epidemiology

Bacterial meningitis is a common disease worldwide. In the United States, approximately 80% of bacterial meningitis cases are caused by the bacteria *Streptococcus pneumonia* and *Neisseria meningitides*, with *Neisseria* predominating in adults less than 45 years of age.[12] The incidence of meningococcal meningitis, caused by *Neisseria meningitides* varies by age group, with rates in neonates and infants as high as

[a] Department of Emergency Medicine, University of Michigan, Taubman Center B1354 SPC #5303, 1500 East Medical Center Drive, Ann Arbor, MI 48109-5303, USA
[b] Department of Neurology, University of Michigan, Taubman Center 1914 SPC #5316, 1500 E. Medical Center Drive, Ann Arbor, MI 48109-5316, USA
* Corresponding author. Department of Emergency Medicine, University of Michigan, Taubman Center B1354 SPC #5303, 1500 East Medical Center Drive, Ann Arbor, MI 48109-5303.
E-mail address: wmeurer@umich.edu (W. Meurer).

Emerg Med Clin N Am 27 (2009) 89–100
doi:10.1016/j.emc.2008.07.004
0733-8627/08/$ – see front matter © 2009 Elsevier Inc. All rights reserved.

400 out of every 100,000 per year and rates in adult in the range of 1 to 2 out of every 100,000 per year.[13,14] The disease appears to occur in males more than females and is most common in the late winter and early spring.[15] Over the past two decades, vaccinations have greatly changed the epidemiology of the disease. The incidence of pneumococcal meningitis caused by *Streptococcus pneumoniae* are beginning to decrease as a result of the routine vaccination of children with heptavalent-pneumococcal conjugate vaccine over the past 8 years.[10] Similarly, the introduction of the *Haemophilus influenza* type b (*Hib*) vaccine has resulted in drastic decreases in cases of *Hib* meningitis and has nearly eradicated disease caused by this pathogen from most of the developed world.[5,7,10,12,16,17]

Pathophysiology

The pathophysiology of meningeal infection has been well studied.[13,18–20] The fact that the three most common pathogens are all encapsulated organisms is not coincidental, and they share features which enable them to invade the host through the upper airway, survive dissemination through the bloodstream, and gain access to the subarachnoid space. The infectious organism first colonizes the nasopharynx, where specialized proteins lead to paralysis of cilia. The host is unable to eradicate the organism and it is able to invade through the mucosa and into the bloodstream. Once bloodborne, the capsule enables the organism to avoid detection and destruction by the complement system. Organisms are then able to cross the blood-brain barrier and proliferate in the CNS. Once in the CNS, inflammation results and is responsible for most of the hallmark symptoms of CNS infection, including fever, meningismus, and altered mental status. Inflammation also increases the permeability of the blood-brain barrier, causing vasogenic edema. Cerebral edema in the nonexpandable cranial vault increases intracranial pressure and results in secondary injury from diminished cerebral perfusion and ischemia.[21]

Other routes of pathogen entry occur, including direct inoculation of the CNS, such as in trauma or surgery, or through direct infection and seeding through parameningeal structures.

Clinical Features

Signs and symptoms

The clinical presentation of patients with meningitis include rapid onset of fever, headache, photophobia, nuchal rigidity, lethargy, malaise, altered mentation, seizure, or vomiting.[22,23] In one study of 493 adult patients with bacterial meningitis, the presence of the "classic triad" of fever, neck stiffness, and altered mental status was present in two-thirds of patients, with fever the most common element, in 95%.[24] Older patients with *S. pneumoniae* meningitis are more likely to have the classic triad.[25] Other studies have shown the classic triad to be less common, with estimates ranging from 21% to 51%.[26,27] All cases studied had at least one of the three signs; the absence of the all components of the classic triad excludes the diagnosis in immunocompetent individuals.[24,28] Immunocompromised individuals are more of a diagnostic challenge, as they may mount none of the classic responses to infection. Meningitis should be in the differential diagnosis of any immunocompromised patient with an infectious disease with altered mental status.[29,30]

Physical examination findings also vary. A careful neurologic examination is important to evaluate for focal deficits and increased intracranial pressure (ICP). Abnormalities in the neurologic examination may necessitate neuroimaging studies. Nuchal rigidity is a common finding. Examination should include assessment for meningeal irritation with Brudzinski's sign (passive flexion of the neck resulting in flexion of the hips and knees) and Kernig's sign (straightening of the knee with a flexed hip resulting in back and neck pain), which are present in 50% of cases.[20] Other important examination findings include purpura or petechia of the skin, which may occur with meningococcemia.

Diagnosis

If the diagnosis of meningitis cannot be ruled out based on history and physical, lumbar puncture (LP) is the procedure of choice for further evaluation.[14,31] In cases of fulminant and clinically obvious meningitis, cerebrospinal fluid (CSF) analysis can serve to speciate causative organisms and guide future antibiotic choice.

In most patients with bacterial meningitis, LP can be safely performed without antecedent neuroimaging. This is not always the case with other CNS pathologies, and so prior head CT to evaluate for mass lesions or increased intracranial pressure may be considered.[32] A general guide for LP without neuroimaging is found in **Box 1**.[32]

The risks of lumbar puncture precipitating brain herniation in meningitis are unclear, but review of case reports and potential pathophysiologic mechanisms has resulted in recommendations to consider LP as relatively contraindicated in patients with "impending" herniation.[33,34] All patients with increased intracranial pressure are at increased risk of herniation and anecdotal data suggests that LP in the presence of increased ICP might precipitate herniation and poor clinical outcomes. In cases where meningitis and increased ICP are suspected, it is reasonable to begin empiric antibiotics and admit the patient for further treatment and work-up, with LP performed at a later time if necessary.[33–36] Recommendations regarding neuroimaging before LP are a moving target and likely will become increasingly controversial in the future (**Box 2**).

Four tubes of CSF, each containing about 1 mL to 2 mL of fluid, should be obtained. Typically, tubes one and four are sent for cell count and differential, tube two for protein and glucose, and tube three for Gram stain and culture. Typical spinal fluid results for meningeal processes are shown in **Table 1**.[37]

Treatment

Treatment of bacterial meningitis has two major goals. The first is the rapid administration of a bactericidal antibiotic with good CNS penetration to treat the neurologic infection, as well as with good tissue penetration to treat possible extra-CNS sources. The second, in select cases, is the use of anti-inflammatory agents to suppress the sequelae of bacterial lysis. Empiric antibiotic choice is based on broad-spectrum coverage of common pathogens. The choice of antibiotics has to be made in consideration of the prevailing pathogens in the locality. Recommendations often include

---

Box 1
Consideration for lumbar puncture without neuroimaging

Age less than 60

Immunocompetent

No history of CNS disease

No recent seizure (less than 1 week)

Normal sensorium and cognition

No papilledema

No focal neurologic defects

Box 2
Controversy in neuroimaging prior to CT

Patients with bacterial meningitis frequently undergo lumbar puncture, and brain herniation is a known complication of fulminant meningitis. Less clear is whether LP can actually precipitate herniation or whether these are simply two epiphenomena associated with the same disease in the same very sick patients. Over the past quarter century, at least 22 cases have been reported of patients with bacterial meningitis who developed brain herniation within hours of having a lumbar puncture. It is not possible to say that herniation could have been prevented in any of these if an LP had not been performed, but there are pathophysiologic reasons to at least speculate that the association may be causal. The practical question confronting the emergency physician is whether a brain CT is required for all patients with suspected meningitis before lumbar puncture to screen for evidence of impending herniation. Given the poor sensitivity of CT scanning for elevated ICP, and the observation that many of the patients with herniation after LP had normal CT scans, there is no simple answer to this question. A reasonable alternative approach is to use clinical evidence of impending herniation to determine the safety of LP. In patients with suspected meningitis and a rapidly deteriorating level of conciousness or brainstem signs (pupillary or respiratory changes), it makes sense to start antibiotics empirically and obtain neuroimaging. The clinician may reasonably defer LP in such patients regardless of whether there is radiographic evidence of midline shift or impending herniation. Although rapid deterioration is possible in any patient with acute bacterial meningitis, those with normal consciousness and intact neurologic examinations are unlikely to have acute herniation precipitated by an LP. If, in fact, lumbar puncture can sometimes precipitate herniation, there is also little evidence that neuroimaging of low-risk patients can identify those likely to have such a complication.

---

ceftriaxone or cefotaxime, and vancomycin for optimal coverage of resistant organisms.[38] Empiric use of vancomycin, however, remains somewhat controversial, with some evidence that harm from drug toxicity in widespread use in children outweighs benefit in the relatively small number of patients that end up having resistant infections.[39] If Listeria is suspected, especially in the very young or old, or those who are immunosupressed, high-dose ampicillin is added. If a penicillin and cephalosporin allergy is present, meropenem or chloramphenicol as well as vancomycin are recommended. Delay in administration of antibiotics has been associated with worsening clinical outcomes. In one study, a 3-hour delay from time of presentation to the hospital to antibiotic administration was independently associated with an increase in 3-month case fatality.[40] It is also important to note that a diagnostic test, whether neuroimaging or CSF testing, must not delay empiric antibiotic therapy.

Table 1
Differential diagnosis of representative CSF analysis parameters

Parameter (normal)	Bacterial	Viral	Neoplastic	Fungal
Opening Pressure (<170 mm)	>300	200	200	300
WBC (<5)	>1000	<1000	<500	<500
% PMNs (0)	>80%	1%–50%	1%–50%	1%–50%
Glucose (>40)	<40	>40	<40	<40
Protein (<50)	>200	<200	>200	>200
Gram Stain (−)	+	−	−	−
Cytology (−)	−	−	+	+

Abbreviations: PMN, polymorphonuclear leukocyte; WBC, white blood cell count.

Anti-inflammatory agents, in theory and in laboratory animals, blunt the massive inflammatory response that CNS infections cause in the enclosed cranial vault and spinal cord.[41] This inflammation is theorized to be responsible for significant negative outcomes despite adequate antimicrobial therapy.[42] Steroids, specifically dexamethasone, have been investigated in numerous meningitis trials, and most data is supportive of its use, at least in adults.[43–45] A Cochrane review including 1,800 patients found a reduction in hearing loss, neurologic sequelae, and mortality in patients treated with dexamethasone as an adjunct to antibiotics.[46] Recent adult and pediatric trials in sub-Saharan Africa did not demonstrate dexamethasone to be efficacious, although the ability to generalize these findings to developed nations and areas without a high prevalence of human immunodeficiency virus seropositivity is unclear.[47,48] Adjuvant corticosteroids in bacterial meningitis is an area of ongoing controversy (**Box 3**).

Current recommendations in adults include the use of dexamethasone, with an initial dose given just before or concurrent with the initial dose of antibiotics, and continuing every 6 hours for 4 days.[14,49] The timing of steroid administration is important and, if administered, they should be given before or concurrent with antibiotics.[14] Pediatric recommendations do not directly address the empiric use of corticosteroids, advocating use only if the organism is known to be *Hib*.[49–51] Because antibiotic administration will almost always precede identification of the causative organism and the incidence of *Hib meningitis* has been reduced dramatically, the utility of this adjunctive therapy in the pediatric age group is unclear.

Antibiotic prophylaxis is recommended for high-risk exposures to patients with *Neisseria* or *Hib meningitis*, with high-risk populations including household contacts, those with exposure to oral secretions, and those who have intubated the patient without a mask. Regimens include single-dose ciprofloxacin or ceftriaxone, or with rifampin, 600 mg every 12 hours for five doses. There is no indication for prophylaxis for exposure to pneumococcal meningitis.[38] Quinolone resistance has been reported to

---

Box 3
Controversy in corticosteroid treatment

Treatment of acute bacterial meningitis with corticosteroids has been controversial for decades, frustrating many practicing clinicians who have seen the pendulum swing back and forth between recommendations to either use or abandon steroids in patients with this highly morbid disease. Although many studies were performed between the 1960s and 1990s, they were generally small and varied in quality. Their validity was also challenged by rapidly changing patterns of illness in the wake of successful *Hib* vaccination programs. Further confusion resulted from various inconsistent findings. For example, some trials reported improvements in survival, while other pediatric trials reported fewer neurologic sequele in survivors but without an actual survival benefit.

Fortunately, several larger, definitive studies have been published in the last 6 years. Trials performed in Europe and Vietnam confirmed the benefit of providing steroids to adult and adolescent patients with definite bacterial meningitis. Two large, high quality trials performed in sub-Saharan Africa in children, however, did not confirm benefit. It is unclear if these studies in developing countries with high rates of HIV ranging from 28% to 90% are directly applicable to practice in the United States. Furthermore, the effect of streptococcal vaccination on the epidemiology of meningitis in children is unclear, and may impact on the utility of steroids.

The best evidence now supports the use of steroids in the treatment of adults with bacterial meningitis, but a confirmatory study in the United States would likely be helpful in consolidating this finding and promoting a change in practice patterns. More pressing is the desperate and clear need for a large randomized, controlled trial of steroid treatment in children with bacterial meningitis in the emergency departments of the developed world.

Neisseria, and this class of antibiotics is no longer recommended for prophylaxis in parts of the United States.[52,53]

Complications

Complications from bacterial meningitis are severe, but with more aggressive antibiotic and critical-care regimens, outcomes are improved. Immediate complications are obvious and devastating, including shock, coma, seizures, respiratory and cardiac arrest, and death.[24] Delayed complications include seizures, paralysis, intellectual deficits, deafness, blindness, bilateral adrenal hemorrhage (Waterhouse-Friderichsen syndrome), and death.[22] Prompt recognition and management of systemic and neurologic complication is crucial to the overall clinical success in these patients.

The fatality rates for pneumococcal meningitis range from 20% to 25%, with higher rates occurring in the elderly and those with other diseases.[54,55] The prognosis appears related to the degree of neurologic impairment on presentation. Overall, 20% to 30% of the survivors of pneumococcal meningitis have some residual neurologic deficit.[22]

The use of antibiotics has decreased the mortality of meningococcal meningitis to less than 20%.[55] Most complications and sequelae are less common that with pneumococcal disease, but the incidence of Waterhouse-Friderichsen syndrome is dramatically higher when meningococcemia is present.[22] The overall mortality rate in community-acquired gram-negative meningitis has been less than 20% since the introduction of the third-generation cephalosporins.[18]

VIRAL MENINGITIS

The common viruses that may cause meningitis include arbovirus, herpes simplex, cytomegalovirus, adenovirus, and HIV.[56] Enteroviruses are most common.[57] As most cases are unreported, precise estimates of incidence are not available, but are thought to be in the range of 11 to 27 individuals per 100,000 people.[58] More cases occur during the summer months.

At times, overlap of CSF findings with early bacterial meningitis or partially treated bacterial meningitis can make diagnosis difficult and can necessitate admission for empiric antibiotics while awaiting culture results. The inability to isolate bacterial pathogens in relation to viral meninigits has led to the term "aseptic meningitis." Numerous decision rules have been proposed to distinguish bacterial from aseptic meningitis, but have not been well validated in broad clinical practice.[59] The clinical course of most of types of viral meningitis is short, benign, and self-limited, and followed by complete recovery. Some infections, like herpes simplex virus (HSV) meningoencephalitis, may have a protacted course (further discussed below).

VIRAL ENCEPHALITIS

Viral encephalitis is an infection and resulting inflammation of the brain parenchyma itself. Although it is different than viral meningitis, the two are often concurrent, and are clinically distinguishable by the presence of neurologic abnormalities in encephalitis.[21]

Epidemiology

Viruses that cause encephalitis include the arboviruses, HSV, herpes zoster virus (HZV), Epstein-Barr virus (EBV), cytomegalovirus (CMV), and rabies. During epidemics, the arboviruses can account for 50% of cases. The four most common have been La Crosse encephalitis, St Louis equine encephalitis, Western equine encephalitis, and Eastern equine encephalitis (EEE).[21] West Nile Virus (WNV) is becoming more prevalent, and had been found in 47 states as of 2003.[60] Encephalitis can lead to significant morbidity and mortality in the extremes of age.

Pathophysiology

Encephalitis-producing viruses enter the host though disease-specific means. The arboviruses (arbo meaning arthropod-borne) are transmitted through mosquito and tick insect vectors. Other agents enter through the respiratory or gastrointestinal tract, through animal bites (ie, rabies), or through blood transfusions or organ transplants.[61] Viral replication invariably occurs outside the CNS, which is then infected through a hematogenous route.[62] Other important viruses, including HSV, rabies, and HZV, reach the CNS through retrograde travel along axons where they have gained access to nerve endings.[62,63]

Once in the brain, the viruses infect neural cells, which can lead to neurologic dysfunction and injury. Particular viruses have affinity for specific CNS cell types, which can affect disease manifestations, such as the affinity of HSV for the temporal lobe.[62]

Clinical Features

As with meningitis, patients with encephalitis may exhibit a wide range of clinical features. With encephalitis, altered levels of consciousness is much more common, including new psychiatric symptoms, cognitive defects, seizures, or focal neurologic deficits.[63] Meningeal irritation including headache, photophobia, and nuchal rigidity is not uncommon. Clinically distinguishing etiologies is difficult because of the large degree of overlap, but again, viral affinity for specific CNS cell types can be useful. For example, temporal lobe seizures are common with HSV, and WNV's affinity for anterior horn cells can result in a Guillain-Barré-like paralysis.[60,64]

Diagnosis

In the emergency department (ED), the focus should be on evaluation and treatment of the immediate life-threatening etiologies, and to rule out other entities that may mimic this presentation, such as bacterial meningitis and subarachnoid hemorrhage. Once these are completed, other tests may help identify the presence of viral encephalitides. LP often shows a picture compatible with aseptic meningitis. CT scan and MRI may show abnormalites.[65–67] The temporal lobes are often affected when HSV is the causative organism.[65,68] There are a number of characteristic EEG findings in encephalitis, especially HSV encephalitis, and EEG is often part of the diagnostic work-up.[69]

Treatment

Only HSV disease has specific therapy available. Acyclovir is capable of improving patient outcome, and is dosed at 10 mg/kg intravenously every 8 hours. Anecdotally, ganciclovir can be used in CMV infections, and pleconaril has shown promise in enteroviral disease.[21,70,71]

Outcomes

Patients with encephalitis necessitate admission, and outcomes are variable depending on etiology. EEE and St. Louis encephalitis generally have high mortality rates and severe neurologic sequelae among survivors.[72] WNV is associated with significant morbidity and morality.[73] Mortality of HSV encephalitis before acyclovir was 60% to 70%, and treatment has now reduced that rate to approximately 30%.[31] Cognitive disability, seizures, and motor deficits are common sequelae seen among survivors.

CENTRAL NERVOUS SYSTEM ABSCESS
Epidemiology

CNS abscesses are found in approximately 2,000 people in the United States annually.[74] Incidence is spread throughout the year, and men are afflicted more than women.[75] Most abscesses have a definable source, which in turn affects the epidemiology of the infection. For example, brain abscess secondary to otitis media occur more frequently in the pediatric population, while those associated with sinusitis are more frequently found among young adults. Immunocompromised patients, including those with HIV and those with solid organ transplant, are also at higher risk. Overall rates have decreased to 0.9 per 100,000 person years, likely because of antimicrobial prophylaxis of immunocompromised populations and treatment of otitis and sinusitis.[74,76]

Pathophysiology

Organisms reach the brain through one of three known routes. Hematogenous spread occurs in one third of cases, contiguous infection from nearby structures in another third, and direct implantation during surgery or trauma in about 10%. The route of infection in the remaining cases is unknown.[21,77] Overall, streptococci are identified in up to 50% of cases.[78] Otogenic infections often contain bacteroides and occur in the temporal lobes or cerebellum.[78,79] Sinus infections lead to brain abscesses in the frontal areas.[78] Rates of postoperative brain abscess was recently found to be 0.2% in a large study, with common organisms being S. aureus and P. acnes.[80] Multiple abscesses usually suggest hematogenous spread, often from endocarditis, intravenous drug abuse, or pulmonary etiologies.[20]

Clinical Features

Patients with intracranial abscess often have a subacute onset of illness and are rarely toxic appearing. Symptoms may progress over a week or more. Fever is present in fewer than half; nuchal rigidity is also rare.[21] Detailed physical examination often reveals the presence of focal deficits and a large number also have papilledema, which is rare with other CNS infections.[76]

Diagnosis

Imaging studies are imperative for diagnosis, with CT scanning being the most commonly used modality.[74] CT scan will often demonstrate hypodense lesions with contrast-enhancing rings, and abscess is one of the few indications for an ED head CT with contrast. MRI will often demonstrate similar findings and is highly sensitive for abscess. LP is inadvisable because of the likely presence of increased ICP and subsequent risk of herniation.[21]

Treatment

ED treatment of intracranial abscess involves initiation of appropriate antibiotics and neurosurgical consultation. Antibiotic choice should take into account likely pathogens (especially anaerobic organisms) as well as CSF penetration, and usually includes a third generation cephalosporin and metronidazole. If the patient is recently postoperative, vancomycin is often added.

Outcomes

With the increased availability of CT scanning, mortality from brain abscess has declined from approximately 50% to less than 20%.[76,77] Common sequelae include seizures (up to 80%), focal motor defects, and continued alterations in mental status.[18]

REFERENCES

1. Vieusseux M. Mémoire sur le maladie qui a régné à Genève au printemps de 1805. Journal of Medical Chirurgical Pharmacology 1805;11:163 [in French].
2. Roos KL. Acute bacterial meningitis. Semin Neurol 2000;20(3):293–306.
3. Vadheim CM, Greenberg DP, Eriksen E, et al. Eradication of *Haemophilus influenzae* type b disease in southern California. Kaiser-UCLA Vaccine Study Group. Arch Pediatr Adolesc Med 1994;148(1):51–6.
4. Madore DV. Impact of immunization on *Haemophilus influenzae* type b disease. Infect Agents Dis 1996;5(1):8–20.
5. Gjini AB, Stuart JM, Lawlor DA, et al. Changing epidemiology of bacterial meningitis among adults in England and Wales 1991–2002. Epidemiol Infect 2006; 134(3):567–9.
6. Albrich WC, Baughman W, Schmotzer B, et al. Changing characteristics of invasive pneumococcal disease in Metropolitan Atlanta, Georgia, after introduction of a 7-valent pneumococcal conjugate vaccine. Clin Infect Dis 2007;44(12): 1569–76.
7. Pollard AJ. Global epidemiology of meningococcal disease and vaccine efficacy. Pediatr Infect Dis J 2004;23(Suppl 12):S274–9.
8. Sharip A, Sorvillo F, Redelings MD, et al. Population-based analysis of meningococcal disease mortality in the United States: 1990–2002. Pediatr Infect Dis J 2006;25(3):191–4.
9. Lexau CA, Lynfield R, Danila R, et al. Changing epidemiology of invasive pneumococcal disease among older adults in the era of pediatric pneumococcal conjugate vaccine. JAMA 2005;294(16):2043–51.
10. Dubos F, Marechal I, Danila MO, et al. Decline in pneumococcal meningitis after the introduction of the heptavalent-pneumococcal conjugate vaccine in northern France. Arch Dis Child 2007;92(11):1009–12.
11. Stedman TL. Stedman's medical dictionary. Philadelphia: Lippincott Williams and Wilkins; 2000.
12. Schuchat A, Robinson K, Wenger JD, et al. Bacterial meningitis in the United States in 1995. Active Surveillance Team. N Engl J Med 1997; 337(14):970–6.
13. Quagliarello V, Scheld WM. Bacterial meningitis: pathogenesis, pathophysiology, and progress. N Engl J Med 1992;327(12):864–72.
14. Fitch MT, van de Beek D. Emergency diagnosis and treatment of adult meningitis. Lancet Infect Dis 2007;7(3):191–200.
15. Fraser DW, Geil CC, Feldman RA. Bacterial meningitis in Bernalillo County, New Mexico: a comparison with three other American populations. Am J Epidemiol 1974;100(1):29–34.
16. Scheifele D, Halperin S, Law B, et al. Invasive *Haemophilus influenzae* type b infections in vaccinated and unvaccinated children in Canada, 2001–2003. CMAJ 2005;172(1):53–6.
17. Peltola H. Worldwide *Haemophilus influenzae* type b disease at the beginning of the 21st century: global analysis of the disease burden 25 years after the use of the polysaccharide vaccine and a decade after the advent of conjugates. Clin Microbiol Rev 2000;13(2):302–17.
18. Lambert HP. Infections of the Central Nervous System. Philadelphia: BC Decker; 1991.
19. Tunkel AR, Wispelwey B, Scheld WM. Bacterial meningitis: recent advances in pathophysiology and treatment. Ann Intern Med 1990;112(8):610–23.

20. Tyler KL, editor. Infectious diseases of the central nervous system. Philadelphia: FA Davis; 1993.
21. Loring K. CNS infections. In: Tintinalli J, editor. Emergency medicine: a comprehensive study guide. New York: McGraw Hill; 2004. p. 1431–7.
22. Geiseler PJ, Nelson KE, Levin S, et al. Community-acquired purulent meningitis: a review of 1,316 cases during the antibiotic era, 1954–1976. Rev Infect Dis 1980; 2(5):725–45.
23. van de Beek D, de Gans J, Tunkel AR, et al. Community-acquired bacterial meningitis in adults. N Engl J Med 2006;354(1):44–53.
24. Durand ML, Calderwood SB, Weber DJ, et al. Acute bacterial meningitis in adults. A review of 493 episodes. N Engl J Med 1993;328(1):21–8.
25. Weisfelt M, van de Beek D, Spanjaard L, et al. Community-acquired bacterial meningitis in older people. J Am Geriatr Soc 2006;54(10):1500–7.
26. Pizon AF, Bonner MR, Wang HE, et al. Ten years of clinical experience with adult meningitis at an urban academic medical center. J Emerg Med 2006;30(4): 367–70.
27. Sigurdardottir B, Bjornsson OM, Jonsdottir KE, et al. Acute bacterial meningitis in adults. A 20-year overview. Arch Intern Med 1997;157(4):425–30.
28. Attia J, Hatala R, Cook DJ, et al. The rational clinical examination. Does this adult patient have acute meningitis? JAMA 1999;282(2):175–81.
29. Aronin SI, Peduzzi P, Quagliarello VJ. Community-acquired bacterial meningitis: risk stratification for adverse clinical outcome and effect of antibiotic timing [see comment]. Ann Intern Med 1998;129(11):862–9.
30. van de Beek D, de Gans J, Spanjaard L, et al. Clinical features and prognostic factors in adults with bacterial meningitis [see comment] [erratum appears in N Engl J Med. 2005 Mar 3;352(9):950]. N Engl J Med 2004;351(18):1849–59.
31. Rowland LP, editor. Merritt's textbook of neurology. 9th edition. Baltimore: Williams & Wilkins; 1995.
32. Hasbrun R, Abrahams J, Jekel J, et al. Computed tomography of the head before lumbar puncture in adults with suspected meningitis. N Engl J Med 2001;345:24.
33. van Crevel H, Hijdra A, de Gans J. Lumbar puncture and the risk of herniation: when should we first perform CT? J Neurol 2002;249(2):129–37.
34. Joffe AR. Lumbar puncture and brain herniation in acute bacterial meningitis: a review. J Intensive Care Med 2007;22(4):194–207.
35. Shetty AK, Desselle BC, Craver RD, et al. Fatal cerebral herniation after lumbar puncture in a patient with a normal computed tomography scan. Pediatrics 1999;103(6 Pt 1):1284–7.
36. Greig PR, Goroszeniuk D. Role of computed tomography before lumbar puncture: a survey of clinical practice. Postgrad Med J 2006;82(965):162–5.
37. Greenlee J. Approach to diagnosis of meningitis: cerebrospinal fluid evaluation. Infect Dis Clin North Am 1990;4:583.
38. Gilbert DN, Moellerng RC, Sande MA, et al. The Sanford guide to antimicrobial therapy 2003. 33rd edition. Portland (OR): Oregon Health Sciences University; 2003. p. 1–150.
39. Buckingham SC, McCullers JA, Lujan-Zilbermann J, et al. Early vancomycin therapy and adverse outcomes in children with pneumococcal meningitis. Pediatrics 2006;117:1688–94.
40. Auburtin M, Wolff M, Charpentier J, et al. Detrimental role of delayed antibiotic administration and penicillin-nonsusceptible strains in adult intensive care unit patients with pneumococcal meningitis: the PNEUMOREA prospective multicenter study. Crit Care Med 2006;34(11):2758–65.

41. Tauber MG, Khayam-Bashi H, Sande MA, et al. Effects of ampicillin and cortico-steriods on brain water content, cerebrospinal fluid pressure, and cerebrospinal fluid lactate levels in experimental penumococcal meningitis. J Infect Dis 1985; 151(3):528.

42. Koedel U, Scheld WM, Pfister HW. Pathogenesis and pathophysiology of pneumococcal meningitis. Lancet Infect Dis 2002;2(12):721–36.

43. Lebel MH, Freij BJ, Syrogiannopoulos GA, et al. Dexamethasone therapy for bacterial meningitis. Results of two double-blind, placebo-controlled trials. N Engl J Med 1988;319(15):964–71.

44. McIntyre PB, Berkey CS, King SM, et al. Dexamethasone as adjunctive therapy in bacterial meningitis. JAMA 1997;278:925.

45. de Gans J, van de Beek D. Dexamethasone in adults with bacterial meningitis. N Engl J Med 2002;347(20):1549–56.

46. van de Beek D, de Gans J, McIntyre P, et al. Corticosteroids for acute bacterial meningitis. Cochrane Database Syst Rev 2007;1:CD004405.

47. Molyneux EM, Walsh AL, Forsyth H, et al. Dexamethasone treatment in childhood bacterial meningitis in Malawi: a randomised controlled trial. Lancet 2002; 360(9328):211–8.

48. Scarborough M, Gordon SB, Whitty CJM, et al. Corticosteroids for bacterial meningitis in adults in sub-Saharan Africa. N Engl J Med 2007;357(24): 2441–50.

49. Tunkel AR, Hartman BJ, Kaplan SL, et al. Practice guidelines for the management of bacterial meningitis. Clin Infect Dis 2004;39(9):1267–84.

50. American Academy of Pediatrics Committee on Infectious Diseases. *Haemophilus influenzae* infections. Redbook 2006;2006(1):310–8.

51. Pneumococcal infections. Redbook 2006;2006(1):525–37.

52. Singhal S. Ciprofloxacin-resistant neisseria meningitidis, Delhi, India. Emerg Infect Dis 2007;13(10):1614.

53. Rainbow J, Boxrud D, Glennen A, et al. Emergence of fluoroquinolone-resistant *Neisseria meningitidis*—Minnesota and North Dakota, 2007–2008. Morb Mortal Wkly Rep 2008;57(7):173–5.

54. Sangster G, Murdoch JM, Gray JA, et al. Bacterial meningitis 1940–79. J Infect 1982;5:245.

55. Wenger JD, Hightower AW, Facklam RR, et al. Bacterial meningitis in the United States, 1986: report of a multistate surveillance study. The Bacterial Meningitis Study Group. J Infect Dis 1990;162(6):1316–23.

56. Specter S, Bendinelli M, Friedman H, et al. Neuropathogenic viruses and immunity. New York: Plenum; 1992.

57. Nowak DA, Boehmer R, Fuchs HH. A retrospective clinical, laboratory and outcome analysis in 43 cases of acute aseptic meningitis. Eur J Neurol 2003; 10(3):271–80.

58. Beghi E, Nicolosi A, Kurland LT, et al. Encephalitis and aseptic meningitis, Olmsted County, Minnesota, 1950–1981: I. Epidemiology. Ann Neurol 1984; 16(3):283–94.

59. Dubos F, Lamotte B, Bibi-Triki F, et al. Clinical decision rules to distinguish between bacterial and aseptic meningitis. Arch Dis Child 2006;91(8): 647–50.

60. Solomon T, Ooi MH, Beasley DW, et al. West Nile encephalitis. BMJ 2003; 326(7394):865–9.

61. Root RK, Sande MA, editors. Viral infections: diagnosis, treatment, and prevention. New York: Churchill Livingstone; 1993. p. 57–71.

62. Johnson RT. The pathogenesis of acute viral encephalitis and postinfectious encephalomyelitis. J Infect Dis 1987;155(3):359–64.
63. Whitley RJ, Soong SJ, Linneman C Jr, et al. Herpes simplex encephalitis. Clinical assessment. JAMA 1982;247(3):317–20.
64. Studahl M, Bergstrom T, Hagberg L. Acute viral encephalitis in adults—a prospective study. Scand J Infect Dis 1998;30(3):215–20.
65. McCabe KK, Tyler KK, Tanabe JJ. Diffusion-weighted MRI abnormalities as a clue to the diagnosis of herpes simplex encephalitis. Neurology 2003;61(7):1015–6.
66. Maschke M, Kastrup O, Forsting M, et al. Update on neuroimaging in infectious central nervous system disease. Curr Opin Neurol 2004;17(4):475–80.
67. Kalita JJ, Misra UUK. Comparison of CT scan and MRI findings in the diagnosis of Japanese encephalitis. J Neurol Sci 2000;174(1):3–8.
68. Kennedy PGE, Chaudhuri A. Herpes simplex encephalitis. J Neurol Neurosurg Psychiatry 2002;73(3):237–8.
69. Lai CW, Gragasin ME. Electroencephalography in herpes simplex encephalitis. J Clin Neurophysiol 1988;5(1):87–103.
70. Redington JJ, Tyler KL. Viral infections of the nervous system, 2002: update on diagnosis and treatment. Arch Neurol 2002;59(5):712–8.
71. Rotbart HA, O'Connell JF, McKinlay MA. Treatment of human enterovirus infections. Antiviral Res 1998;38(1):1–14.
72. Anderson JR. Viral encephalitis and its pathology. Curr Top Pathol 1988;76: 23–60.
73. Centers for Disease Control and Prevention. West Nile virus activity—United States, October 30–November 5, 2003. MMWR Morb Mortal Wkly Rep 2003; 52(44):1080.
74. Calfee DP, Wispelwey B. Brain abscess. Semin Neurol 2000;20(3):353–60.
75. Mathisen GE, Johnson JP. Brain abscess. Clin Infect Dis 1997;25(4):763–79 [quiz 780–1].
76. Carpenter J, Stapleton S, Holliman R. Retrospective analysis of 49 cases of brain abscess and review of the literature. Eur J Clin Microbiol Infect Dis 2007;26(1): 1–11.
77. Yang SY. Brain abscess: a review of 400 cases. J Neurosurg 1981;55(5):794–9.
78. Wispelwey B, Scheld WM. Brain abscess. Semin Neurol 1992;12(3):273–8.
79. Small M, Dale BA. Intracranial suppuration 1968–1982: a 15-year review. Clin Otolaryngol Allied Sci 1984;9(6):315–21.
80. McClelland S, Hall WA. Postoperative central nervous system infection: incidence and associated factors in 2,111 neurosurgical procedures. Clin Infect Dis 2007; 45(1):55–9.

Emergency Treatment of Status Epilepticus: Current Thinking

Dan Millikan, MD, Brian Rice, MD, Robert Silbergleit, MD*

KEYWORDS

- Seizure • Status epilepticus • Benzodiazepines
- Anticonvulsants • Emergency treatment

Current thinking about the acute treatment of status epilepticus (SE) emphasizes a more aggressive clinical approach to this common life-threatening neurologic emergency. Three aspects of this approach are discussed here: initiating first-line therapy more rapidly, accelerating progression to second-line therapy when needed, and considering nonconvulsive SE more often.

Most patients who present to the emergency department (ED) with seizures have self-limited episodes. Care in such patients is primarily focused on determining the cause of the new-onset or breakthrough seizure, and the patient's clinical outcome is generally determined by the underlying pathology precipitating the seizure. Most often, patients with isolated seizures have a good prognosis.

In contrast, SE is a true medical emergency, with substantial morbidity and mortality. The prognosis in patients who have SE depends not only on the underlying disease but on successful treatment of the seizures from clinical and electrographic perspectives. In several large patient series, the overall 30-day mortality rate of patients who had generalized convulsive status epilepticus (GCSE) ranged from 19% to 27%.[1–3] Mortality was higher in those patients who remained in GCSE for an hour or longer[2,4] and in patients older than 65 years of age or those in whom seizures were precipitated by anoxia.[2] Furthermore, mortality may be three times higher in patients who have SE with subtle convulsive or nonconvulsive SE, in whom seizure activity is only clearly distinguished from other causes of unresponsiveness electroencephalographically.[3]

Complications of prolonged seizures include indirect systemic problems arising from the convulsive state and direct neuronal cellular injury resulting from excitotoxicity itself. The convulsive state can cause impaired ventilation and subsequent pulmonary aspiration, cardiac dysrhythmias, and derangements of systemic metabolic and autonomic function. Neuronal injury results from molecular cascades of injury involving excitatory neurotransmission, calcium-mediated injury, membrane and

---

Department of Emergency Medicine, University of Michigan Neuro Emergencies Research, 24 Frank Lloyd Wright Drive, Lobby H, Suite 3100, PO Box 381, Ann Arbor, MI 48106, USA
* Corresponding author.
E-mail address: robie@umich.edu (R. Silbergleit).

Emerg Med Clin N Am 27 (2009) 101–113
doi:10.1016/j.emc.2008.12.001

mitochondrial failure, and protease-mediated damage in the cytosol and the nucleus. These processes result in immediate neuronal loss and delayed programmed cell death.[5] More rapid termination of SE protects against neuronal injury in experimental SE in laboratory animals and is associated with better patient outcomes in clinical observation.

In experimental models, benzodiazepines are more effective and work more quickly when given earlier after the onset of seizure. These effects may result from changes in γ-aminobutyric acid (GABA) receptor subunit composition that are associated with decreased pharmacoresponsiveness to subsequent treatment with benzodiazepines when effective treatment is delayed by several minutes.[6] Rapid termination of seizures also prevents kindling effects demonstrated in animal models, in which seizures become more refractory to subsequent treatment as the duration of seizures increases.[7] Rapid treatment may also prevent the neuronal cell injury and loss that occurs with increasing duration of seizures attributable to duration-dependent cytokine-mediated effects.[8]

Clinical data also demonstrate that the duration of SE is associated with more frequent death and unfavorable neurologic outcomes.[2,4,9,10] Although many of these data concern long durations of SE lasting hours or days, data also suggest that differences of as little as a few minutes in seizure duration are associated with differences in outcome. Patients found in SE by paramedics who had termination of their seizures before arrival to the ED had an intensive care unit (ICU) admission rate of 32% as compared with 73% in patients whose seizures persisted on arrival to the ED.[11] In a randomized trial, patients who had SE treated with lorazepam or diazepam in the field by paramedics had mortality rates at hospital discharge of 7.7% and 4.5%, respectively, which was less than half the mortality rate of 15.7% for patients in whom benzodiazepines were given only after arrival in the ED.[11]

This review considers four concepts that can accelerate effective treatment of SE. These include (1) updating the definition of SE to make it more clinically relevant, (2) consideration of faster ways to initiate first-line benzodiazepine therapy in the prehospital environment, (3) moving to second-line agents more quickly in refractory status in the ED, and (4) increasing detection and treatment of unrecognized nonconvulsive SE in comatose neurologic emergency patients.

NEW DEFINITION OF STATUS EPILEPTICUS

Developing the sense of urgency required to treat SE more rapidly begins by clarifying and refining the relevant terminology. Traditionally, SE has been clinically defined as seizures persisting or recurring without a return to consciousness for an extended period, usually 30 minutes or more. More recently, the rationale for these durations has been challenged and a more useful clinically relevant definition of greater than 5 minutes of unrelenting seizure has been advanced.

Ideally, the definition of SE would be mechanistic rather than dependent on clinical duration of symptoms. Despite substantial research and advances in the field, however, the pathophysiology of SE is still poorly understood and a mechanistic definition is not yet tenable. Until the physiology of SE is better understood, it has to be operationally defined based on a somewhat arbitrarily selected duration of seizure activity. The longer durations traditionally used to define SE were selected based on assumptions about underlying pathophysiology that are now known not to be true rather than on any kind of clinical relevance. Defining SE as seizure persisting for longer than 5 minutes is theoretically and practically advantageous for several reasons.

First and foremost, seizing for 30 minutes or more is a long time. The implication of the traditional definition of SE is that until a patient has been seizing for this duration, his or her seizure is prognostically consistent with the kind of brief self-limited seizure associated with good clinical outcomes. That is, by saying that a patient has SE only after 30 minutes of seizure activity is to imply that any seizure lasting for a shorter time than this is benign. Empirically, this is not true. Data from continuous electroencephalographic (EEG) monitoring indicate that the average length of a benign, self-limited, adult generalized tonic-clonic seizure (including pre-tonic-clonic, tonic, and clonic phases) is just longer than a minute and only rarely persists beyond 2 minutes. Patients with seizures that last more than 5 minutes are not likely to improve spontaneously. Consequently, most of these patients are more similar to those with seizures of 30 to 60 minutes' duration than they are to patients with benign seizures of less than 5 minutes' duration. Thus, the new definition is better at discriminating prognostically.

Second, the definition of SE should be relevant to the clinical treatment required. Whereas benign self-limited seizures can be treated by merely supporting the patient and preventing injury, patients who have SE require treatment with anticonvulsants. It is untenable to allow a patient to seize for longer than 30 minutes before providing anticonvulsants. The definition of status should be relevant to emergency treatment and care and consistent with clinical practice. This is in contrast to current practice patterns, which support treatment of prolonged seizures long before 30 minutes.

Finally, the traditional definition of SE is rooted in some outdated speculation about the onset of neuronal injury. Earlier definitions used cutoffs of longer than 30 minutes, partially because this is when histopathologic changes in the brain were first reliably noted after experimental SE in some older laboratory studies. Although understanding of the physiology of neuronal injury in SE remains incomplete, it is now clear by using more sensitive assays of neuronal loss that cellular injury can start much earlier, within minutes of seizure onset. Ultimately, a definition of SE that distinguishes seizures without neuronal injury from seizures with such injury would be desirable; however, for now, a useful definition based on mechanism is not clinically feasible. Certainly, the traditional definition does not work mechanistically.

In response to these concerns about the conventional definition of SE, Lowenstein proposed a new definition for the disorder, which was published in *Epilepsia* in 1999.[12]

Generalized convulsive status epilepticus in adults and older children (greater than 5 years old) refers to greater than 5 minutes of a continuous seizure, or two or more discrete seizures between which there is incomplete recovery of consciousness.

Defining status in this way allows us to recognize short-lasting seizures as relatively benign events not necessarily requiring emergent treatment and gives us strong grounds to treat longer lasting seizures aggressively as true emergencies necessitating strong pharmacologic intervention. Better defining the problem is the first step toward faster and more effective treatment.

PREHOSPITAL TREATMENT OF STATUS EPILEPTICUS

Advanced emergency medical services (EMS) systems offer the opportunity to provide early pharmacologic interventions to patients with acute conditions in which minutes matter. Laboratory and clinical data suggest that SE is one of those conditions. As noted previously, laboratory data from experimental SE suggest that treatment is most likely to terminate seizures successfully when delivered shortly after the onset of ictus. Changes in the GABA subunit that binds benzodiazepines and other allosteric modulators occur rapidly during prolonged seizures. As a result, seizures are most responsive to benzodiazepine treatment within the first 10 minutes after seizure on-set.[6] Later treatments have a lower rate of terminating seizures or require higher doses to achieve the same rate. Laboratory data also show that longer seizures cause kin-dling effects in which the brain reorganizes itself in response to excess neural activa-tion, resulting in increased susceptibility to further seizures.[7] Treating SE faster has the potential to reduce not only the risks of the immediate seizure but the risk for having more frequent seizures in the future. Theoretically, paramedics have the opportunity to treat patients who have SE at a time when benzodiazepines are most likely to be effective at stopping seizures and at a time when stopping the seizures is likely to optimize patients' outcomes.

Clinical trial data have confirmed that early treatment of prehospital SE is effective. The benefit of initiating prehospital treatment for SE was demonstrated in the Preho-spital Treatment of Status Epilepticus (PHSTE) trial. In this randomized clinical trial (RCT), patients with out-of-hospital seizures lasting longer than 5 minutes who were treated by San Francisco EMS were randomized to receive intravenous diazepam, lor-azepam, or placebo. The study showed that significantly more patients given diaze-pam or lorazepam had early termination of their seizures before arrival in the ED, as compared with patients given placebo.[11] Although the difference was not quite statis-tically significant, 30% of the placebo group died in the hospital or were discharged with a new neurologic deficit, as compared with 23% of patients given lorazepam or diazepam by paramedics. Furthermore, patients whose seizures were terminated before ED arrival had a much lower rate of ICU admission (32%) than patients who were still seizing on arrival (73%; $P<.001$).

These data confirm that prehospital treatment of SE by paramedics is effective and suggest that early termination of seizures is clinically beneficial. Therefore, research efforts must now identify the optimal drug and route of administration for use in the prehospital environment. In the PHTSE trial, there was a strong trend toward higher efficacy and decreased seizure time with intravenous lorazepam as compared with in-travenous diazepam (**Fig. 1**).[11] The PHTSE investigators concluded that lorazepam should be recommended over diazepam as the first-line medication for prehospital treatment of SE. This recommendation is consistent with current in-hospital manage-ment of SE, but there are practical difficulties with lorazepam that have prevented its widespread adoption by EMS systems.

Although lorazepam is the most common first-line anticonvulsant used for initial treatment of SE in the ED, it is relatively heat labile compared with other benzodiaze-pines like diazepam or midazolam, which have long shelf lives at ambient tempera-tures. It is recommended that lorazepam be kept in refrigerated storage or that it be frequently restocked, which makes it prohibitive for most EMS systems, especially smaller systems that may only infrequently use the medication. Lorazepam is also ap-proximately 10% more expensive than equipotent doses of diazepam or midazolam, adding an incremental financial burden to struggling EMS systems.[13]

Another limitation of lorazepam is that it requires intravenous administration. In con-trast, other more lipophilic benzodiazepines can be administered by transmucosal or intramuscular routes. The use of such alternative routes of administration is particu-larly attractive in the prehospital treatment of SE, because gaining intravenous access can be challenging in patients with violent convulsions. Trying to start an intravenous line in convulsing patients also increases the risk for needlestick injuries to para-medics. Furthermore, starting and securing an intravenous line can be time-consum-ing and can delay the treatment of SE. One commonly used alternative to intravenous benzodiazepines in SE is the rectal administration of diazepam, which comes in a gel formulation labeled for this purpose. Unfortunately, the effectiveness of diazepam

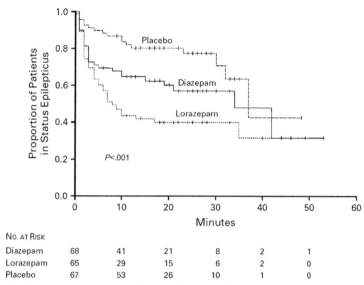

No. at Risk

Diazepam	68	41	21	8	2	1
Lorazepam	65	29	15	6	2	0
Placebo	67	53	26	10	1	0

Fig. 1. Benzodiazepines were more effective than placebo at terminating seizures before ED arrival in the PHTSE trial.[11] Kaplan-Meier curves compare the durations of out-of-hospital SE after treatment with lorazepam, diazepam, or placebo. Tick marks indicate censoring of data. The curves were significantly different from one another by the log-rank test (P<.001).

given by this route is quite limited in patients who have SE.[14] In addition, rectal administration can be physically challenging in the acutely seizing patient and is often socially undesirable for patients and paramedics. Lorazepam can also be given across mucus membranes by means of rectal, nasal, or buccal administration. Despite some encouraging preliminary data,[14] however, a large, recently completed, randomized controlled trial demonstrated that lorazepam was not effective when given by transmucosal routes to patients who have SE.[15]

Among the possible alternatives to intravenous administration, paramedics are likely most familiar with giving intramuscular injections. The intramuscular route has received increased attention in recent years. A handful of preliminary clinical trials, predominantly performed in children, have evaluated the safety and efficacy of this route using midazolam.[16–20] Unlike diazepam and lorazepam, midazolam is highly lipophilic and is rapidly absorbed after intramuscular administration. Midazolam administered intramuscularly has been consistently shown to produce serum levels at 80% of peak levels within 5 minutes of administration. Clinically, midazolam given intramuscularly or across mucus membranes is as effective as intravenous diazepam at terminating seizures in patients who have SE and is more rapid when one takes into account the time needed to start an intravenous line **(Fig. 2)**.[21]

Midazolam may likely be a better agent for the prehospital treatment of SE, even though it is not labeled by the US Food and Drug Administration (FDA) for that purpose. It does not have the storage or cost problems of lorazepam, and in preliminary trials, it seems to be more effective than diazepam. It is effective when given intramuscularly or by other transmucosal routes. Many EMS systems are already carrying midazolam for other indications, so medics are often familiar and comfortable with its use. Informal estimates suggest that many systems, as many as 30% of those in the United

Review: IV diazepam versus IM/IN midazolam for treatment of seizure
Comparison: 01 Effectiveness of IM/IN MDZ as compared to IV DZP
Outcome: 01 Termination of seizure

Study or sub-category	IV Diazepam n/N	IM/IN Midazolam n/N	RR (fixed) 95% CI	Weight %	RR (fixed) 95% CI
Chamberlain	11/13	12/13		8.99	0.92 [0.69, 1.21]
Lahat	24/26	23/26		17.23	1.04 [0.87, 1.25]
Rainbow	23/62	23/45		19.96	0.73 [0.47, 1.12]
Mahmoudian	28/35	21/35		15.73	1.33 [0.97, 1.83]
Shah	54/65	45/50		38.10	0.92 [0.80, 1.07]
Total (95% CI)	201	169		100.00	0.97 [0.86, 1.09]

Total events: 140 (IV Diazepam), 124 (IM/IN Midazolam)
Test for heterogeneity: Chi² = 6.87, df = 4(P = 0.14), I² = 41.8%
Test for overall effect: Z = 0.54 (P = 0.59)

0.5 0.7 1 1.5 2
Favors IM/IN MDZ   Favors IV DZP

Review: IV diazepam versus IM/IN midazolam for treatment of seizures
Comparison: 01 Effectiveness of IM/IN MDZ as compared to IV DZP
Outcome: 02 Time to seizure control

Study or sub-category	IV DZP N	IV DZP Mean (SD)	IM/IN MDZ N	IM/IN MDZ Mean (SD)	WMD (fixed) 95% CI	Weight %	WMD (fixed) 95% CI
Chamberlain	11	11.20 (3.60)	13	7.80 (4.10)		3.51	3.40 [0.32, 6.48]
Lahat	26	8.00 (4.10)	26	6.10 (3.60)		7.58	1.90 [-0.20, 4.00]
Shah	65	4.20 (2.30)	50	1.60 (0.90)		88.91	2.60 [1.99, 3.21]
Total (95%CI)	102		89			100.00	2.58 [2.00, 3.15]

Test for heterogeneity: Chi² = 0.68, df = 2 (P = 0.71), I² = 0%
Test for overall effect: Z = 8.74 (P < 0.00001)

-10 -5 0 5 10
Favors IM/IN MDZ   Favors IV DZP

Fig. 2. Meta-analysis of clinical studies of intramuscular (IM) or intranasal (IN) midazolam versus intravenous (IV) diazepam in patients who have SE demonstrates similar efficacy in terminating seizures within 10 minutes of administration but more rapid termination of seizures if time to obtain intravenous access is considered. CI, confidence interval; df, degrees of freedom; RR, relative risk.

States, have already switched from diazepam to midazolam as first-line treatment for SE. Protocols for its use vary, but the preferred dosing is likely to be 2 mg/kg for children and 10 mg for adults.

Despite increasing use and encouraging preliminary data, the use of intramuscular midazolam in patients who have SE has not yet been proved safe and effective in a large RCT. Such a trial, comparing intramuscularly administered midazolam in an autoinjector with intravenously administered lorazepam in the prehospital treatment of patients who have SE, has been organized and funded by the National Institutes of Health and is scheduled to commence soon at sites throughout the United States.

In the meantime, intramuscular midazolam remains a promising treatment for patients treated by paramedics for out-of-hospital SE. It has become an increasingly popular but currently unproved option for prehospital providers.

EMERGENCY DEPARTMENT TREATMENT OF STATUS EPILEPTICUS

Historically, a variety of treatments have been used empirically for the initial treatment of SE. At the turn of the nineteenth century, anecdotal treatment successes were reported with a combination of oral morphine, potassium bromide, and chloral hydrate. Later, in the early twentieth century, several case series described favorable results with a variety of agents, including phenobarbital in 1912, paraldehyde in the 1940s, and phenytoin in the 1950s. The benzodiazepine diazepam was first described as a treatment for SE in the early 1960s.[22]

In 1983, Leppik and colleagues[23] performed a randomized double-blind trial comparing the effectiveness of diazepam, 10 mg, versus lorazepam, 4 mg, as initial therapy for SE. If these initial doses did not terminate seizures within 10 minutes, an identical second dose was administered. Lorazepam was successful in 89% (29 of 37) of subjects, and diazepam was successful in 76% (25 of 33) of subjects. Although this difference was not statistically significant in this trial, lorazepam gained in popularity and has become the preferred first-line therapy for SE. After additional unpublished studies performed by the manufacturer demonstrated the superiority of lorazepam to diazepam, and the superiority of lorazepam at 4-mg doses to lorazepam at 1- or 2-mg doses, the FDA approved lorazepam for the treatment of SE in adults in 1997.[24]

Other large studies of first-line therapy in SE followed. The Veterans Affairs Status Epilepticus Cooperative Study was a large RCT that compared four distinct treatments for SE in subjects with a variety of seizure types.[3] Although the analysis of this trial was complex, the investigators concluded that intravenous lorazepam at 0.1 mg/kg was at least as effective and easier to use than the alternative treatments, which included phenobarbital, diazepam plus phenytoin, and phenytoin. Subsequently, the previously discussed PHTSE trial was the only study of first-line therapy to include a control group, and it confirmed the efficacy of benzodiazepines in general and lorazepam in particular. Results are pending from two large trials of lorazepam in pediatric patients, one of which has recently ended and one of which is ongoing.[15,25]

Although there are sufficient data to support the use of intravenous lorazepam as the preferred first-line agent for the treatment of SE in the ED, similar data are not available to suggest the best agents and the optimal timing of therapy for refractory SE in patients who do not respond to first-line therapy. Comprehensive protocols for the treatment of SE therefore depend heavily on expert opinion and vary considerably among individuals and institutions but tend to be based on the recommendations of the Epilepsy Foundation of America's Working Group on Status Epilepticus as published in 1993.[26] This group recommended the sequential use of benzodiazepine, phenytoin, phenobarbital, and then general anesthesia, which is well known today. The general layout of this conventional sequence is shown in **Fig. 3**.

Over the past 15 years, however, the wisdom of this conventional sequence has been challenged. Data from the Veterans Affairs Status Epilepticus Cooperative Study in particular raised questions about the incremental efficacy of each step in this

A
Conventional protocol

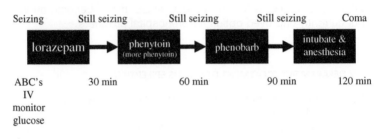

B
Consolidating treatment steps

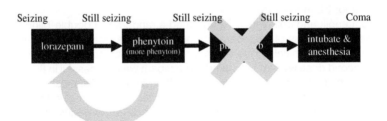

C
Proposed accelerated protocol

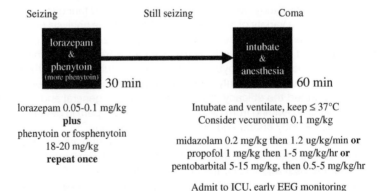

Fig. 3. Protocols for ED treatment of SE. Graphic presentation of a conventional protocol (*A*), potential ways to consolidate steps in such a protocol (*B*), and an example of an accelerated treatment protocol (*C*).

sequence. In patients who had overt GCSE and failed initial first-line therapy, the addition of a second drug resulted in only 5% additional successful treatments. Further, addition of a third drug, regardless of the agent used, added only 2.3% more. Although each added treatment step provided only marginal benefit, the sequential approach consumed substantial time and prolonged the interval until burst suppression under general anesthesia for those with refractory SE, a step that was successful in an additional 23% of subjects. The infusion time of agents varied in the Veterans Affairs Status Epilepticus Cooperative Study, from approximately 16 minutes for phenobarbital to 42 minutes for diazepam and phenytoin in addition to time given after delivery of each agent to see if the treatment was going to work.[3,22]

Given the observations that the intermediate steps of the conventional sequence have limited added value and increased awareness of the importance of earlier termination of seizures, changes to the conventional treatment sequence have been proposed (see **Fig. 3**). A new accelerated protocol has been proposed in which the previously sequential steps of lorazepam and phenytoin are now stacked and given simultaneously and in which phenobarbital has been omitted. In principle, this accelerated strategy should allow more aggressive treatment of patients who have SE and should reduce the delay to the induction of pharmacologic coma (thereby improving the outcomes) in those with the most refractory seizures. Clinical research to determine if this is true in practice is still required.

The optimal agent for general anesthesia in SE is unclear. The most widely described agents are pentobarbital, midazolam, and propofol, and high-quality comparative efficacy data for each are not available. Nonrandomized retrospective data from a series of 20 patients found similar efficacy and outcomes with propofol and midazolam.[27] A systematic review suggested substantial efficacy of any of these agents if titrated to burst suppression on continuous EEG monitoring in the ICU setting.[28]

Current thinking about the treatment of SE in the ED suggests using an accelerated treatment strategy to terminate seizures as quickly as possible. Close cooperation and early collaboration with specialists in neurologic critical care are required to make such protocols seamless and to transition patients rapidly from ED care to ICU care when seizures are refractory.

NONCONVULSIVE STATUS EPILEPTICUS IN THE EMERGENCY DEPARTMENT

GCSE is usually easily recognized in the ED. Nonconvulsive status epilepticus (NCSE, also sometimes called "subtle GCSE") is less familiar to emergency physicians and far less clinically obvious. Although generally considered a rare condition, more extensive use of continuous EEG monitoring in the ICU (and occasionally in the ED) now suggests that seizures without convulsions are more common than previously estimated. Nonconvulsive seizures and NCSE can be (1) the source of continued coma after GCSE, (2) the cause of unexplained coma, or (3) a supplemental cause of coma in patients with other known central nervous system pathologic findings. Appreciation of this diagnosis suggests the possibility that continuous EEG monitoring in the ED may offer new opportunities to intervene and improve the outcomes of patients with neurologic emergencies.

At the turn of the nineteenth century, investigators described the phenomenon of generalized protracted seizure activity. Clark and Prout, in a series of articles published in 1903 and 1904 in the *American Journal of Insanity* entitled "Status Epilepticus: A Clinical and Pathological Study in Epilepsy," provided a detailed description of the clinical presentations and pathologic correlations of patients who have GCSE.[29–31] Significantly, in many cases of overt GCSE, they described the evolution of convulsions over time to more subtle focal twitching of the eyelids or face, nystagmus, extremity or trunk twitching, and then to no discernible movement whatsoever. With the advent of EEG, the phenomenon of persistent EEG ictal activity with subtle or absent motor findings has been called NCSE or subtle GCSE.[32] NCSE may be a manifestation of previously diagnosed epilepsy, or it can be a new-onset form of seizure in the acute phase of any number of different neurologic insults, including hypoxic-ischemic encephalopathy, stroke, traumatic brain injury (TBI), and meningitis.[33–35]

Emergency physicians should be familiar with two general subtypes of NCSE that have been colorfully described by Fujikawa[36] as the "walking wounded" and the "ictally comatose." The former are more accurately termed *absence status epilepticus* and *complex partial status epilepticus*. Patients who have these conditions may present with a variety of altered mental status. They may present with acute or subacute confusional states that may include alterations in alertness, memory, judgment, or language. Emotional lability is common, and patients who have these forms of NCSE are often misdiagnosed as having psychiatric diagnoses or substance abuse problems. The presence of motor automatisms may clue the astute clinician in the ED that EEG is warranted. Ultimately, these are difficult diagnoses, and they are rarely confirmed in the emergency setting. Furthermore, it is not yet established that rapid treatment of these forms of SE is an important modifier of clinical outcomes in these patients. The potential adverse effects of drugs and interventions in SE, such as loss of airway reflex, aspiration pneumonia, and hypotension, need to be taken into consideration. Awareness of complex partial SE can help the emergency physician to diagnose this unusual cause of altered mental status, in addition to triggering early consultation with the neurology service to establish a definite diagnosis and effective treatment plan collaboratively.

Far less is known about ictally comatose patients, but this condition may potentially be far more important for emergency physicians to diagnose. These patients present with acute coma or obtundation from ongoing generalized electrographic seizure activity and are thought to have the same systemic pathologic changes and excitotoxicity seen in GCSE. Patients who have this form of NCSE have a poor prognosis, and rapid interventions to terminate seizures in these patients are likely to improve patient outcomes, although there are few data to answer this question directly. Most cases of NCSE are diagnosed in patients who have GCSE and remain unconscious after cessation of convulsive activity. It is also frequently considered in patients who have known epilepsy or similar risk factors and are found unconscious for no other apparent reason. Patients like these are not uncommon in neurologic critical care but seem to be rarer in the ED.

Recent evidence, however, suggests that the ictally comatose patient may be far more common in the ED than previously suspected. Increased use of continuous EEG monitoring in the ICU setting has revealed a remarkably high incidence of secondary nonconvulsive seizures and NCSE complicating other forms of primary acute neurologic injury. Vespa and colleagues[37] reported that 22% of patients with moderate to severe TBI had intermittent seizure activity on continuous EEG monitoring and that 6% had NCSE. Furthermore, patients who had TBI and NCSE had 100% mortality. In a small study of patients who had acute stroke, 27% of those with ischemic subtype and 28% of those with hemorrhagic subtype were found to have NCSE. In those who had ischemic stroke, NCSE was associated with a threefold increase in mortality that was independent of infarct size, and in those with hemorrhagic stroke, NCSE was associated with risk for clinical deterioration and edema that was independent of the hematoma size.[35,38] Evidence that NCSE is a modifiable complication in acute brain injury and not just a marker of more severe injury comes from observations in patients who have subarachnoid hemorrhage (SAH). In 2007, Little and colleagues[39] analyzed 389 patients who had spontaneous SAH, 11 (3%) of whom developed NCSE. Once detected, control of NCSE was obtained in 4 patients, 2 of whom survived and had good neurologic outcomes, whereas 7 patients in whom NCSE could not be controlled all died.

NCSE seems to be a common and potentially important modifier of neurologic outcome. Furthermore, it seems to be an early development after the onset of injury. Up to 71% of cases of NCSE are diagnosed within the first hour of continuos EEG monitoring when that monitoring is begun in the ICU.[34] Further work is needed to determine how many patients with these acute problems have NCSE while still in the ED and whether interventions in the ED successfully improve outcome.

In the current setting, in which patient safety is paramount, the use of EEG in the ED not only can direct early appropriate interventions to those patients with seizures but can spare patients presenting with EEG-negative seizure-mimicking episodes the potential adverse effects of seizure therapies. Surveillance for NCSE in patients with other primary acute neurologic emergencies requires the ability to monitor EEG continuously in the ED. Although this modality is generally unavailable in most EDs, the feasibility of extending such monitoring to the ED has been demonstrated.[33] More widespread implementation in EDs is likely to rely on the development and validation of systems that are different from those used in the ICU. ED systems are likely to need to use a relatively limited montage and to have reliable analytic routines for automatic detection of prolonged seizure activity.

Such technologies have outstanding potential and are currently being commercially designed and tested. Clinical observational studies and clinical trials are needed to confirm the frequency of NCSE in the ED and to confirm that treatment of NCSE, when detected, can improve patient outcomes.

SUMMARY

Current thinking is that the emergency treatment of SE should be faster and more aggressive. More clinical trials are needed to determine the optimal management of patients who have SE, but many important lessons can be implemented in the meantime:

- Patients with unrelenting seizures lasting longer than 5 minutes are at increased risk for poor clinical outcomes and should be defined as having SE.
- Midazolam given intramuscularly is a promising treatment in the prehospital setting to treat seizures. A clinical trial is underway to establish its role as a first-line option for the treatment of SE, especially in the prehospital setting.
- In the ED, treatment of SE can be accelerated by delivering lorazepam and phenytoin simultaneously on arrival and progressing directly to general anesthesia if the first-line agents fail and seizures continue. This approach needs to be balanced by the potential adverse effects that these interventions may have on patients.
- In the future, the ability to monitor EEG continuously in the ED is likely to identify a substantial number of patients who have NCSE, providing an opportunity to intervene and potentially improve patient outcomes.

The management of patients who have SE requires emergency physicians and specialists in neurologic critical care to work together to provide care that is initiated early and maintained appropriately as patients progress from the ED to the ICU.

REFERENCES

1. Logroscino G, Hesdorffer DC, Cascino G, et al. Short-term mortality after a first episode of status epilepticus. Epilepsia 1997;38:1344–9.
2. Towne AR, Pellock JM, Ko D, et al. Determinants of mortality in status epilepticus. Epilepsia 1994;35:27–34.
3. Treiman DM, Meyers PD, Walton NY, et al. A comparison of four treatments for generalized convulsive status epilepticus. Veterans Affairs Status Epilepticus Cooperative Study Group. N Engl J Med 1998;339:792–8.
4. Sloan E. The treatment of status epilepticus patients in the emergency setting. In: Wasterlain C, Treiman D, editors. Status epilepticus: mechanisms and management. Cambridge: MIT Press; 2006. p. 597–605.
5. Lowenstein DH, Alldredge BK. Status epilepticus. N Engl J Med 1998;338:970–6.
6. Kapur J, Macdonald RL. Rapid seizure-induced reduction of benzodiazepine and Zn2+ sensitivity of hippocampal dentate granule cell GABAA receptors. J Neurosci 1997;17:7532–40.
7. Morimoto K, Fahnestock M, Racine RJ. Kindling and status epilepticus models of epilepsy: rewiring the brain. Prog Neurobiol 2004;73:1–60.
8. Ravizza T, Vezzani A. Status epilepticus induces time-dependent neuronal and astrocytic expression of interleukin-1 receptor type I in the rat limbic system. Neuroscience 2006;137:301–8.
9. Maegaki Y, Kurozawa Y, Hanaki K, et al. Risk factors for fatality and neurological sequelae after status epilepticus in children. Neuropediatrics 2005;36:186–92.
10. Holtkamp M, Othman J, Buchheim K, et al. Predictors and prognosis of refractory status epilepticus treated in a neurological intensive care unit. J Neurol Neurosurg Psychiatr 2005;76:534–9.
11. Alldredge BK, Gelb AM, Isaacs SM, et al. A comparison of lorazepam, diazepam, and placebo for the treatment of out-of-hospital status epilepticus. N Engl J Med 2001;345:631–7.
12. Lowenstein DH, Bleck T, Macdonald RL, et al. It's time to revise the definition of status epilepticus. Epilepsia 1999;40:120–2.
13. Moore Medical Supplies. Available at: www.mooremedical.com. Accessed August 10, 2008.
14. Appleton R, Sweeney A, Choonara I, et al. Lorazepam versus diazepam in the acute treatment of epileptic seizures and status epilepticus. Dev Med Child Neurol 1995;37:682–8.
15. National Institutes of HealthRandomized trial comparing 3 routes of delivering lorazepam to children. The National Institutes of Health, 2008. Available at: http://www.clinicaltrials.gov/ct2/show/NCT00343096 Accessed August 10, 2008.
16. Chamberlain JM, Altieri MA, Futterman C, et al. A prospective, randomized study comparing intramuscular midazolam with intravenous diazepam for the treatment of seizures in children. Pediatr Emerg Care 1997;13:92–4.
17. Mahmoudian T, Zadeh MM. Comparison of intranasal midazolam with intravenous diazepam for treating acute seizures in children. Epilepsy Behav 2004;5:253–5.
18. Rainbow J, Browne GJ, Lam LT. Controlling seizures in the prehospital setting: diazepam or midazolam? J Paediatr Child Health 2002;38:582–6.
19. Shah I, Deshmukh CT. Intramuscular midazolam vs intravenous diazepam for acute seizures. Indian J Pediatr 2005;72:667–70.
20. Lahat E, Goldman M, Barr J, et al. Comparison of intranasal midazolam with intravenous diazepam for treating febrile seizures in children: prospective randomised study. BMJ 2000;321:83–6.

21. Silbergleit R, Lowenstein DH, Barsan W. Comparing routes of benzodiazepine administration in the initial emergency treatment of persistent seizures: a meta-analysis. In: The Fourth Mediterranean Emergency Medicine Congress. Sorrento, Italy; September 16–18, 2007.

22. Faught E, DeGiorgio C. Generalized convulsive status epilepticus: principles of treatment. In: Wasterlain C, Treiman D, editors. Status epilepticus: mechanisms and management. Cambridge: MIT Press; 2006. p. 481–9.

23. Leppik IE, Derivan AT, Homan RW, et al. Double-blind study of lorazepam and diazepam in status epilepticus. JAMA 1983;249:1452–4.

24. Food and Drug Administration NDA approval package 18140/S003. Available at: www.fda.gov. Accessed October 10, 2008.

25. National Institutes of Health. Efficacy and safety study comparing lorazepam and diazepam for children in the emergency department with seizures. National Institutes of Health, 2008. Available at: http://clinicaltrialsgov/ct2/show/NCT00621478. Accessed August 10, 2008.

26. Treatment of convulsive status epilepticus. Recommendations of the Epilepsy Foundation of America's Working Group on Status Epilepticus. JAMA 1993;270:854–9.

27. Prasad A, Worrall BB, Bertram EH, et al. Propofol and midazolam in the treatment of refractory status epilepticus. Epilepsia 2001;42:380–6.

28. Claassen J, Hirsch LJ, Emerson RG, et al. Treatment of refractory status epilepticus with pentobarbital, propofol, or midazolam: a systematic review. Epilepsia 2002;43:146–53.

29. Clark LP, Prout TP. Status epilepticus: a clinical and pathological study in epilepsy (part 1). Am J Psych 1903;60:291–306.

30. Clark LP, Prout TP. Status epilepticus: a clinical and pathological study in epilepsy (part 2). Am J Psych 1904;60:645–98.

31. Clark LP, Prout TP. Status epilepticus: a clinical and pathological study in epilepsy (part 3). Am J Psych 1904;61:81–108.

32. Alldredge BK, Treiman DM, Bleck T, et al. Treatment of status epilepticus. In: Engel J, Pedley T, editors. Epilepsy: a comprehensive textbook. Philadelphia: Lippincott-Raven; 2007. p. 1357–63.

33. Bautista RE, Godwin S, Caro D. Incorporating abbreviated EEGs in the initial workup of patients who present to the emergency room with mental status changes of unknown etiology. J Clin Neurophysiol 2007;24:16–21.

34. Claassen J, Mayer SA, Kowalski RG, et al. Detection of electrographic seizures with continuous EEG monitoring in critically ill patients. Neurology 2004;62:1743–8.

35. Jordan KG. Emergency EEG and continuous EEG monitoring in acute ischemic stroke. J Clin Neurophysiol 2004;21:341–52.

36. Fujikawa D. The two faces of electrographic status epilepticus: the walking wounded and the ictally comatose. In: Wasterlain C, Treiman D, editors. Status epilepticus: mechanisms and management. Cambridge: MIT Press; 2006. p. 109–12.

37. Vespa PM, Nuwer MR, Nenov V, et al. Increased incidence and impact of nonconvulsive and convulsive seizures after traumatic brain injury as detected by continuous electroencephalographic monitoring. J Neurosurg 1999;91:750–60.

38. Waterhouse EJ, Vaughan JK, Barnes TY, et al. Synergistic effect of status epilepticus and ischemic brain injury on mortality. Epilepsy Res 1998;29:175–83.

39. Little AS, Kerrigan JF, McDougall CG, et al. Nonconvulsive status epilepticus in patients suffering spontaneous subarachnoid hemorrhage. J Neurosurg 2007;106:805–11.

Enhancing Community Delivery of Tissue Plasminogen Activator in Stroke Through Community – Academic Collaborative Clinical Knowledge Translation

Phillip A. Scott, MD

KEYWORDS

- Knowledge translation • Stroke
- Thrombolytic • Treatment • tPA

Improving the clinical outcomes of stroke patients depends on the adoption of proven new therapies throughout the broader medical community. Approximately 1% of stroke patients in community settings are receiving tissue plasminogen activator (tPA) therapy 12 years after US Food and Drug Administration approval.[1–7] Data suggest substantial improvement in treatment rates is possible, with current treatment rates considerably less than estimates of eligible patients[8] and those reported in optimized stroke care systems.[1,9,10]

Knowledge translation, the process by which the results of clinical investigations are adopted by clinicians and incorporated into routine practice, is important but often overlooked. The development and implementation of educational interventions to motivate physicians and other health care providers, along with health care organizations, to learn the principles of acute stroke care has been declared a high-priority objective of the National Institute of Neurological Disorders and Stroke (NINDS).[11] Ideally, knowledge translation is a collaborative process involving physicians practicing in a community environment and academic physicians who have special expertise.

Given the societal burden of stroke, the demonstrated efficacy of thrombolytic therapy, and the potential of even more aggressive stroke treatment strategies

This work was supported by Grant No. R01 NS50372 from the National Institutes of Health.
Department of Emergency Medicine, University of Michigan, 24 Frank Lloyd Wright Drive, Lobby H, Suite 3100, P.O. Box 381, Ann Arbor, MI 48106-0381, USA
E-mail address: phlsctt@med.umich.edu

(glycoprotein 2B3A inhibitors, intra-arterial thrombolysis, mechanical clot disruption, and so forth) effective and efficient methods to enhance physician delivery of acute stroke care must be realized. Failure to do so marginalizes the impact of proven and future stroke therapies.

This article reviews the history of tPA use in stroke as a case study of a breakdown of knowledge translation in emergency medicine. It briefly reviews knowledge translation concepts and theory and explores practical community–academic collaborative methods based on these tenets to enhance acute stroke care delivery in the community setting.

KNOWLEDGE TRANSLATION
Definition

Simply put, knowledge translation reflects the movement of new findings from the laboratory setting, to clinical investigation, to common usage. A widely cited knowledge translation definition was published in 2004 by the Canadian Institutes for Health Research, in which knowledge translation was defined as "the exchange, synthesis and ethically sound application of knowledge within a complex system of interactions among researchers and users—to accelerate the capture of the benefits of research...through improved health, more effective services and products, and a strengthened health care system."[12]

The Institute of Medicine has subdivided the knowledge translation process based on obstacles to implementation of new science. The first subdivision (T1) represents the challenges in research moving from basic science to human investigational studies. The second subdivision (T2) represents those difficulties in moving successful therapies from clinical trials into common practice and health decision making.[13] This second area represents the focus of this article.

With the emergency department positioned as both the portal through which many patients are admitted and the place routine health care is often provided, the premature, late, or non-adoption of new medical science has profound implications with respect to patient and societal health and efficient use of resources.

Even for less critical injuries, the failure to adopt proven strategies carries cost. Lang and colleagues[14] examined the knowledge translation failure of implementation and adherence to the Ottawa Ankle Rules. Even though the rules are well validated, extensively published, low-risk, and provide estimated cost savings of (US) $3,145,910 per 100,000 patients evaluated, use of the tool remains limited.

The recognition of the importance of knowledge translation in emergency medicine was underscored in 2007 by the Academic Emergency Medicine consensus conference to establish a research agenda on knowledge translation and evidence uptake.[15]

Theories of Behavioral Change

Physicians and other health care providers have traditionally relied on persuading individuals to change through "informational power" (sharing facts about disease processes) and "expert power" (using professional credentials to impress others with the potential effectiveness of the prescribed behavioral change).[16] Such approaches, however, do not fully mesh with current theories of health promotion and behavior change theories.

Knowledge seems to be necessary, but insufficient alone, for behavioral changes to take place. Although differences exist among the predominant behavioral change theories (Health Belief Model, Theory of Reasoned Action, Subjective Expected Utility Theory, and Social Cognitive [Learning] Theory) several core concepts are common among them: perceived probability of disease occurring, perceived severity of disease, perceived effectiveness of the behavioral change in decreasing the probability and severity of disease, and perceived cost of (or barriers to) enacting the change.[17-19] Some component of self-efficacy, the perception of one's own ability to successfully take action, has also been incorporated into most current theories of health promotion behavior. Multilevel interventions may thus be required to change practice behavior.

KNOWLEDGE TRANSLATION OF TISSUE PLASMINOGEN ACTIVATOR USE IN STROKE
Bench to Bedside

In 1995, the NINDS rt-PA Stroke Study Group demonstrated the efficacy of tPA (alteplase) in the treatment of acute stroke.[20] This study elaborated one set of clinical conditions under which use of tissue plasminogen activator resulted in a favorable outcome. These conditions included: (1) use of a lower dose than given in myocardial infarction, (2) administration within 3 hours of symptom onset (defined as the time the patient was last normal), and (3) excluded patients who had blood pressure in excess of 185/110 at the time of treatment.

Of the 624 patients in the trial, 43% of treated patients were neurologically intact at 3 months as compared with 27% of placebo-treated patients. These results were statistically and clinically significant and durable out to 1 year.[21] Mortality was 17% in treated patients and 21% in the placebo group, a difference that was not statistically significant. Patients who had intracranial hemorrhages were included in the benefit analysis and the higher rate of good outcomes occurred despite an increased risk for symptomatic hemorrhage (6.4% versus 0.6%) within 36 hours in the treatment group.

Seven other randomized, double blind, placebo-controlled clinical trials evaluating use of thrombolytic drugs in stroke have been published.[22-27] These evaluated significantly different clinical trial conditions, including different drugs and doses, time windows of treatment, and subject inclusion/exclusion criteria. These studies were unsuccessful in defining a set of conditions in which treatment was efficacious. **Table 1** provides a summary of these studies and their differences with the NINDS trial.

Bedside to Clinical Practice

Governmental and professional approval
Based on the NINDS rt-PA stroke study, the US Food and Drug Administration approved tPA for use in acute stroke in 1996. Canada's Health Products and Food Branch subsequently approved its use in 1999, and the European Agency for the Evaluation of Medicinal Products followed in 2002.[28]

Numerous professional and community organizations have endorsed tPA use in stroke, including: the American Academy of Neurology,[29] American College of Chest Physicians, American Heart Association/American Stroke Association,[30] Canadian Stroke Consortium, National Stroke Association, and multiple others. Additionally, the National Institutes of Health (NIH) sponsored national symposia on promoting treatment of acute stroke in 1997[31] and again in 2002.[32]

Notably absent from the list of endorsing professional organizations was emergency medicine representation. In 1996 the American College of Emergency Physicians (ACEP) agreed "with reservations" to the new stroke guidelines.[33] In 2002, ACEP issued a policy statement indicating "intravenous t-PA may be an efficacious therapy" but that "there is insufficient evidence to endorse the use of t-PA…when systems are not in place to ensure that…NINDS guidelines…are followed." The decision to use tPA

Table 1
Summary of major differences in thrombolytic trials in stroke

Study	Location	Drug	Dose	Time (h)	Exclusion Criteria
ATLANTIS A[24] (1991–1993)	United States	rt-PA	0.9 mg/kg (max: 90 mg)	0–6	Blood pressure
NINDS[20] (1991–1994)	United States	rt-PA	0.9 mg/kg (max: 90 mg)	0–3 (1:59)[a]	Blood pressure
MAST-I[22] (1991–1995)	Italy, United Kingdom, Portugal	streptokinase	1.5 million U	0–6	
ECASS 1[26] (1992–1994)	Europe	rt-PA	1.1 mg/kg (max: 100 mg)	0–6 (4:24)[a]	CT evidence of early infarct; age
MAST-E[23] (1992–1994)	France, United Kingdom	streptokinase	1.5 million U	0–6 h (4:36)[b]	Mild stroke
ASK Trial[25] (1992–1994)	Australia	streptokinase	1.5 million U	0–4 (3:28)	Age; minor stroke
ATLANTIS B[21] (1993–1998)	United States	rt-PA	0.9 mg/kg (max: 90 mg)	3–5 (4:36)[b]	Blood pressure; age
ECASS 2[27] (1996–1998)	Europe , Australia, New Zealand	rt-PA	0.9 mg/kg (max: 90 mg)	0–6	Blood pressure; CT evidence of early infarct; age

Abbreviations: ASK, Australian streptokinase study; ATLANTIS, alteplase thrombolysis for acute noninterventional therapy in ischemic stroke; ECASS, European cooperative acute stroke study; MAST, multicenter acute stroke trial.
[a] Mean.
[b] Median time onset-to-treatment.

"should begin at the institutional level."[34] The American Academy of Emergency Medicine issued a position statement in 2002 to address issues of medical-legal liability. Their position paper stated, "Debate on the safety, efficacy and applicability of tPA has limited its widespread use. Nonetheless, an increasing number of liability suits are emerging against physicians for not administering tPA…" and stated that there was insufficient evidence to classify tPA use in stroke as a standard of care.[35]

In an effort to address these concerns and statistical criticisms of the original study, the NIH/NINDS sponsored an independent, external reanalysis of the study data by personnel not connected with the original trial. The reviewers had access to the entire data set and reported their findings at the 2003 Society of Academic Emergency Medicine annual meeting. This presentation, and subsequent publication of the results, confirmed the original findings of benefit to tPA-treated patients in the trial.[36]

Post-approval studies
Over the past decade, multiple post-approval studies and smaller case series have reported on tPA use in various settings. The following summarizes major studies geographically.

United States The Standard Treatment with Alteplase to Reverse Stroke (STARS) study was a prospective, 57-center study involving 24 academic and 33 community hospitals in the United States. A total of 389 stroke patients consecutively treated with tPA between 1997 and 1998 were evaluated.

This study found a 30-day mortality of 13% and a very favorable outcome (defined as a modified Rankin Score [mRS] of ≤ 1) of 35%, with 43% being functionally independent (mRS ≤ 2). The rate of symptomatic intracranial hemorrhage within 3 days of treatment was 3.3% (95% CI: 1.8% to 5.6%), lower than that reported in the NINDS trial. Protocol deviations occurred in 33% of patients, with treatment beyond the 3-hour window, premature use of anticoagulants (within 24 hours), and excessive pre-tPA blood pressures identified in 13%, 9%, and 7% of patients, respectively.[37]

Canada The Canadian federal government, as a condition of drug licensure, mandated the Canadian Alteplase for Stroke Effectiveness Study (CASES). This study was a prospective treatment registry with patient follow-up 90 days after stroke to assess the safety and effectiveness of alteplase in the context of routine care.

A total of 1135 sequentially treated stroke patients were included from 60 centers between 1999 and 2001, representing an estimated 84% of all treated ischemic stroke patients in the country over that period. Excellent clinical outcomes occurred in 37% and symptomatic intracranial hemorrhage was identified in 4.6% (95% CI: 3.4% to 6.0%) of patients. Again, these compare favorably to the results of the NINDS data.[38] The median time from stroke onset to treatment was 155 minutes (interquartile range: 130–175). Protocol violations occurred in 14%, with treatment beyond 3 hours, elevated INR, and inappropriate dosing of tPA (>90 mg) accounting for 86%, 8%, and 5% of violations, respectively.

European Union The largest post-approval study to date was the 2007 observational Safe Implementation of Thrombolysis in Stroke Monitoring Study (SITS-MOST) from the European Union.[28] As with CASES, this study was mandated by the European Union as a condition of drug licensure to assess the safety profile of alteplase in routine clinical practice when administered within 3 hours of symptom onset.

SITS-MOST was a prospective, open, multicenter study of tPA use in the European Union (as of 2002) in addition to Norway and Iceland. A total of 285 centers participated. Comparisons were made between the 6483 patients treated according to European Union label eligibility criteria and pooled data from the NINDS, European Cooperative Acute Stroke Study (ECASS) I and II, and Alteplase Thrombolysis for Acute Noninterventional Therapy in Ischemic Stroke (ATLANTIS) stroke studies. European Union label eligibility limited treatment to patients between 18 and 80 years of age and NIH stroke scale scores of 25 or less.

Participating centers were required to have a stroke unit or similar monitoring capability for tPA-treated patients and clinical responsibility for patient management was held by a neurologist or stroke physician who had experience. Furthermore, the label eligibility requirement of the study limited a complete exploration of the clinical use of tPA because there were no data on treatment eligibility violations or its effects, profoundly limiting the usefulness of these data.

In this large cohort, mortality within 3 months was 11.3% (95% CI: 10.5 to 12.1). The symptomatic intracranial hemorrhage rate was 7.3% (95% CI: 6.7% to 7.9%), slightly higher than that reported in the NINDS trial. In comparing new treatment centers against experienced treatment centers, there was no increase in intracranial hemorrhages. A small difference in 90-day mortality was identified, with new centers reporting 13.3% (95% CI: 14.1 to 21.1) versus 10.6% (95% CI: 9.8 to 11.6) for experienced centers, although both values were less than the comparison pooled results.

Very favorable outcome (mRS≤1) occurred in 39% of patients, identical to the NINDS study. Functional independence (mRS≤2) was achieved in 54.8% (95% CI: 53.5% to 56.0%). The authors concluded that alteplase, when used within 3 hours of stroke onset and according to label eligibility requirements, had a safety profile at least as good as that seen in published clinical trials.[28]

Current use

The proportion of stroke patients potentially or actually eligible for thrombolytic therapy has been reported to range from 0% to 22%.[39] Despite the accumulating evidence, however, intravenous tPA therapy remains unused in the vast majority of patients.

Data from Cleveland indicate 17% of ischemic stroke patients were admitted within 3 hours of symptom onset, yet only 1.8% received intravenous tPA.[3] Data from the multistate Paul Coverdell Stroke Registry indicate only 3% of patients received some form of fibrinolytic therapy (either intravenous or intra-arterial).[6] The nationwide (United States) inpatient sample data taken between 1999 and 2004 indicate thrombolytic use occurred in 1.1% (95% CI: 0.95 to 1.32) of ischemic stroke hospitalizations. Some 70% of the approximately 1000 hospitals reporting data never used thrombolysis for stroke. In those that did, the mean annual number of treatments was three.[7] These data support previous reports of usage rates of 1% to 3% in the community setting.[1–5,7]

Contrasting these figures to the cardiac data is revealing. In the National Registry of Myocardial Infarction, of the 240,989 patients who had myocardial infarction between 1990 and 1993, 35% received thrombolytic therapy.[40]

Although stroke is typically more difficult for the layperson to recognize and often a greater diagnostic challenge for the clinician, it is reasonable to believe treatment of a larger proportion of patients who have ischemic stroke is possible. A veteran stroke service in Houston, Texas reported 8.7% of admitted patients who had symptoms of cerebral ischemia were treated with intravenous tPA from 1996 to 2000. Impressively, during the study's final 6 months, 12.9% of all patients were treated with intravenous tPA.[9]

Based on the proportion of eligible patients, the use of thrombolytics in the setting of myocardial infarction, and the experience of well-developed thrombolytic stroke teams, it seems possible to increase stroke treatment beyond current levels.

Emergency medicine acceptance of acute stroke treatment

A 1999 survey reporting the perceptions of 701 postgraduate year 1 to 4 emergency medicine residents regarding tPA use found 73% considered their knowledge of thrombolytic therapy very good or somewhat good and 88% indicated they would personally use tPA if they had a stroke. Only 4% indicated they would not use tPA in stroke under any circumstances.[41]

This relative enthusiasm of emergency physicians in training contrasts with the findings of a subsequent 2005 survey from 1105 ACEP members that found extremely limited acceptance of acute treatment of stroke with tPA. In this survey, 45% (95% CI: 37% to 44%) reported they were not likely to use tPA for stroke even in the ideal setting. Of those, 65% reported their reluctance was attributable to perceived risk for symptomatic intracranial hemorrhage, 23% to lack of benefit, and 12% to both.[42]

KNOWLEDGE TRANSLATION BARRIERS IN STROKE
Understanding Barriers in Knowledge Translation

Cabana and colleagues[43] published a comprehensive assessment of the barriers to physician adherence to clinical practice guidelines and organized them into a theoretical framework. This framework details their interplay and their effects on physician knowledge, attitudes, and behavior—the domains necessary to influence for successful knowledge translation (**Fig. 1**).

Specific barriers that may limit successful adoption of new guidelines include those influencing awareness, familiarity, and physician agreement with new recommendations on treatment. Other barriers include the belief that a given practitioner can deliver a new therapy (self-efficacy), that a particular outcome following treatment will be observed (outcome expectancy), and overcoming the inertia of previous practice. External barriers, those issues outside the control of the clinician, may prevent new treatment guideline adoption.

The implications of this framework indicate successful knowledge translation depends on addressing unique barriers at the level of the individual physician and his or her practice environment. What is effective in improving treatment behavior in one hospital setting thus depends on the presence, type, and intensity of barriers faced, and may not be successful in another.

Barriers to Tissue Plasminogen Activator Use

An examination of the barriers to improving the treatment of stroke patients is found within the NINDS proceedings on the rapid identification and treatment of acute stroke. The authors noted "Delivery systems for acute stroke hospital care are relatively primitive compared with systems for...cardiac care...and the recent approval of intravenous tPA has exposed these deficiencies and mandates changes in the hospital care system."[31] The lack of a systems-based approach is of major concern to emergency physicians as stated earlier in the ACEP policy on tPA use in stroke.

In a systematic review of barriers to tPA delivery in acute stroke, Kwan and colleagues[39] noted the following specific barriers within the health care system to thrombolytic delivery: emergency medical system (EMS) triage of stroke as an emergency, emergency department failure to triage stroke as an emergency, delays in

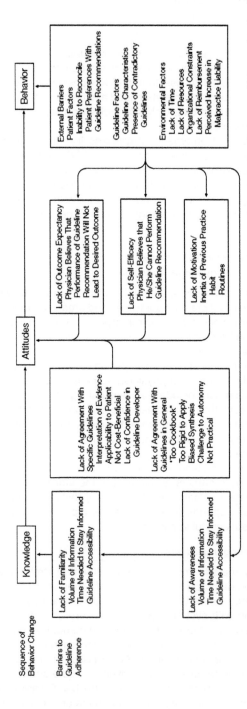

Fig. 1. Barriers to physician adherence to practice guidelines in relation to behavior change. (*From* Cabana MD, Rand CS, Powe NR, et al. Why don't physicians follow clinical practice guidelines? A framework for improvement. JAMA 1999;282(15):1458–65; with permission.)

neuroimaging, inefficient processes of emergency stroke care, and physician uncertainty in administering tPA. Other identified barriers included inadequate training in stroke for doctors.

Identifying Site-Specific Stroke Barriers

Interventions to improve knowledge translation would therefore ideally target those barriers found in a specific hospital/emergency department environment. Because behavioral change to increase tPA use in stroke needs to occur within a complex organization (a hospital) the organization's barriers to treatment must be identified, understood, and addressed for education to succeed and behavior to change. The following techniques may prove useful in identifying site-specific barriers to stroke care.

Qualitative assessment

Qualitative research derives information from observation, interviews, or verbal interactions to establish insights into the perceptions or experiences of a target group. Analysis is interpretative and subjective and statistical tests are not used. These techniques are commonly used in marketing and social science and may be beneficial in evaluating barriers to knowledge translation at the staff level. Methods used include focus groups and structured interviews and allow understanding of participant knowledge, attitudes, behavior, and motivations.

Prior qualitative work found physician characteristics are related to specific barriers. In research examining adherence to national guidelines for asthma management, senior physicians mentioned lack of agreement with medication recommendations and the inertia of previous prescribing patterns as barriers, whereas younger physicians described lack of confidence in dosing or recognizing contraindications. Both groups mentioned time limitations.[44]

Understanding potential group differences can enhance the effectiveness of local knowledge translation processes in acute stroke care and other disease conditions. Although an extensive review of the use of qualitative techniques in identifying stroke barriers is beyond the scope of this article, additional detail on may be found in a review by Muerer and colleagues.[45]

Site resource assessment

Although health care providers possess strong internal motivation to assimilate new information to improve the quality of care they provide, this desire must compete against numerous environmental barriers. An assessment of physical resources and tools considered necessary in the delivery of tPA in stroke is reasonable. One suggested listing of these is in **Box 1**.

CHANGING STROKE PRACTICE: T2 KNOWLEDGE TRANSLATION

In general, six methods are available at the local level to influence physician behavior change: education, audit/feedback mechanisms, physician champion development, administrative intervention, and financial incentives/disincentives.[46]

Education

Post-training education of physicians typically consists of traditional continuing medical education (CME) offered as a didactic lecture to enhance physician knowledge. Although successful in increasing knowledge, the impact of traditional CME alone in changing physician behavior is extremely limited.[47,48] Randomized controlled trials of the impact of interactive CME (small group, workshops, training sessions, and so

---

Box 1
Suggested elements of acute stroke treatment resource assessment

Clinical policy/procedure for acute stroke care/tPA use

Triage screening tool (Cincinnati Prehospital Stroke Scale; Los Angeles Prehospital Stroke Scale)

Neurology on-call list

Specialized stroke response paging system

Stroke-specific documentation templates for nursing staff and physicians

Rapid laboratory result access

Rapid CT scanner access

Rapid CT interpretation access

Preprinted nursing orders for stroke patients

Blood pressure management guidelines for pre- and post-tPA treatment

tPA use inclusion/exclusion checklists

Pre-printed tPA use in stroke informed consent (with outcome expectation, mortality and intracerebral hemorrhage complication information preprinted)

tPA weight-based dosing worksheets

NIH stroke scale scoring forms

Rapid drug access (pharmacy or emergency department stock)

Preprinted admission or transfer orders for post-tPA patients

---

forth) and mixed CME (elements of both didactic and interactive formats) have found greater success.[49–55] It seems unlikely that stroke education, offered in isolation by standard CME processes, will substantially alter stroke treatment behavior, but it is an important first step.

Repetition seems important in increasing the likelihood of success in educational efforts. In a review of randomized controlled trials of CME, Davis and colleagues[49] found 7 of 10 repetitive CME interventions (most using two sessions in a series) had a positive effect compared with 2 of 7 singular interventions.

The use of simulation training (eg, mock stroke codes) and immediately available treatment protocols provide alternate delivery vehicles for educational content and may address other barriers to behavior change also.

Ideally, the educational topics presented, whether addressed in CME-type forums or in other educational methods, address major categories of barriers (lack of awareness, familiarity, agreement, self-efficacy, outcome expectancy, inertia, or external barriers) previously identified. Suggestions for educational methods and content to address specific barriers follow and are summarized in **Table 2**.

Improving awareness

Physicians may be unaware of recommendations for the use of tPA by the NINDS and other national groups (American Heart Association, American Academy of Neurology). Conversely, they may adhere to more limited recommendations by the American Academy of Emergency Medicine or ACEP. Information in a lecture format describing the various recommendations, their development process, and the data used to develop them, could address this barrier.

Table 2 Content suggestions for barrier-specific continuing medical education sessions	
Identified Barriers	**Suggested CME Content**
Awareness of tPA use guidelines	Compare/contrast guideline development, data, and recommendations American Heart Association/American Stroke Association ACEP AAEM
Agreement with guidelines	Review guideline source data and post-approval data NINDS tPA stroke study NINDS tPA stroke study reanalysis STARS, CASES, SITS-MOST Cleveland use of tPA
Self-efficacy for tPA delivery	Neurologic assessment skills Use of the NIH stroke scale Emergency physician diagnostic accuracy in stroke Use of local treatment protocols Promotion of electronic aids Simulation training: mock stroke codes
Outcome expectancy	Review NINDS short- and long-term outcome data Review other post-approval study outcome data Use local cases for evaluation and review
Overcoming inertia of previous practice	Use of local opinion leaders in interactive session Present local performance data Create competition between stakeholders Review coding/billing process and financial impact
External barriers	Identify and address hospital-specific external barriers

Increasing agreement

Within emergency medicine, considerable debate has emerged regarding agreement on the appropriateness of the use of tPA in stroke. In a BMJ article a member of the board of the ACEP was quoted, "Leaders in emergency medicine are raising significant scientific, ethical and implementation issues [regarding the use of tPA in stroke]." This stance has been heatedly debated within the emergency medicine community.[56–58]

The essential issues voiced in these debates regard concern over lack of efficacy, lack of effectiveness (that results obtained by highly motivated researchers are not replicable in the general community), and limited system support for tPA delivery.

To address efficacy issues, a discussion examining the results of the original NINDS trial and the subsequent independent re-examination of the data[36] is suggested. To address issues regarding effectiveness, a review of the post-approval studies noted earlier and use of tPA by emergency physicians is recommended.[59–64]

Enhancing self-efficacy

Self-efficacy is the belief that one can actually perform a behavior. Increased self-efficacy is associated with increased likelihood that a person will perform a given behavior.[65] The delivery of tPA in stroke requires confidence in: patient evaluation skills; knowledge of indications and contraindications of tPA use; expected risks and benefits for discussion with patients/families; and the ability to coordinate care between the emergency department, radiology, and neurology. A mixed continuing education session targeting specific topics of interest could include reviewing neurologic assessment skills using case-presentation formats; the use of the NIH stroke scale as an evaluation tool; or reviewing emergency physician accuracy in stroke diagnosis. Other methods to address self-efficacy barriers include clinical guideline development and stroke simulation scenarios.

Stroke treatment protocol development Clinical practice guidelines, another form of physician education, have only limited effects on changing physician behavior[66–68] often because of multiple barriers, internal and external, to the behavior change process. The advantages of these tools, however, are standardization of processes and care, low cost, and ease of distribution. Such tools are readily available and can be in paper or electronic format. One popular tool includes a palm-based application for stroke assessment and treatment available for free from the Foundation for Emergency Research in Neurologic Emergencies at http://www.ferne.org.

Simulation: mock stroke codes Code situations are medical or surgical emergencies requiring an immediate response for successful patient resuscitation. Patients presenting with acute stroke eligible for tPA represent a neurologic code situation. Even in large hospitals, however, a stroke code represents a low-frequency event, more akin to pediatric/neonatal resuscitation codes than the more familiar cardiac or trauma codes.

Previous work indicates residents in medical training fail to maintain knowledge and skills learned in advanced life support courses and often return to their pretraining level within 12 months.[69,70] In a study of resident physician performance in pediatric codes, Cappelle and Paul[71] found a series of code simulations resulted in significant improvements in residents' perceived need for additional knowledge, confidence in their performance, and motor skills in arrest situations.

It is reasonable, therefore, to conduct mock acute stroke codes for training purposes. Planning of such events should incorporate nursing and physician input using the framework advocated by Funkhouser and colleagues[72] in the development of multidisciplinary mock codes. This framework uses an assessment-planning-implementation-evaluation process and designates various on-site responsibilities before the session, enhancing buy-in of the process from key personnel.

Frequency of mock code delivery should be based on baseline stroke volume, staff turnover, perceived need, performance, and other factors. Codes should be interdisciplinary, be conducted with advance notification to staff to enhance participation and reduce anxiety, use pre- and postcode sessions to review objectives and evaluate performance, use actual supplies (protocols, triage tools, communication assets), and include usual nursing and physician charting.

Code scenarios should incorporate a vignette, role-played by a staff member (or use a mannequin), with a directing facilitator, who provides baseline presentation information. It is recommended to test multiple scenarios over time and include patients both eligible and ineligible for tPA. The actions of the participants determine the outcome of the vignette and the observer/reviewer should have pre-established detailed instructions for critical decision points. Codes typically last 15 to 30 minutes and should be followed by a 10-minute debriefing to allow participants to evaluate their success and areas for improvement.

Increasing outcome expectancy

Outcome expectancy is the belief that performing a behavior will lead to the desired outcome. High outcome expectancy is associated with an increased likelihood of performing a behavior.[65] Emergency physicians are often insulated from the ultimate outcome of treated patients. These factors potentially contribute to low outcome expectancy within the emergency department. Reviewing outcome data from the NINDS trial and the post-approval studies noted previously could potentially address this issue. Promoting case reports of local treatment success is an additional method.

Removing inertia of previous practice

The inertia of previous practice because of habit, custom, or previous training is also a barrier to the use of tPA in stroke. To address this element, physicians have to be motivated to move from a precontemplative stage to an action stage in readiness to change practice. Techniques that may help overcome the inertia of previous practice include performance feedback and opinion leader beliefs.[73] Incorporating the use of local opinion leaders and discussing performance may aid in creating a competitive performance environment between stakeholders.

Reducing external barriers

These barriers represent impediments to tPA delivery in stroke beyond the physician's immediate control. Educational interventions to address barriers of this nature should focus on planned or completed modifications to eliminate specific barriers. These may often be of an administrative or resource nature. A frequent issue of this type is real-time access to neurology/stroke-specialist consultation.

Given the low-frequency, high-morbidity, high-mortality nature of ischemic stroke—in addition to the highly variable presentations of stroke patients and stroke mimics—the promotion of local consultation systems to provide real-time access to stroke specialists may remove the perception of isolation of the treating emergency physician and improve physician-to-physician knowledge transfer. Not all facilities have access to local neurologists or stroke experts, however.

The use of simple telephone consultation with tertiary stroke centers has been shown to substantially increase stroke treatment volume and be a safe, practical, and effective method of extending care to hospitals with limited resources.[74,75] More sophisticated telemedicine applications, combining real-time audio and video transmission with remote patient evaluation and management by stroke specialists, are also available and have proven feasible and effective in expanding acute stroke treatment.[76,77] Limitations of these techniques include the need to establish relationships in advance with remote consultants and processes to access them in a time-critical setting.

Education summary

In conclusion, educational efforts to enhance physician stroke education should deliver content in a learner-centered, active format that addresses the learner's needs and is simultaneously engaging and reinforcing.[49] The multiple sequencing of events within a single day and over multiple months offers a "learn-work-learn" opportunity in which education may be translated into practice.

Audit/Feedback

Audit and feedback interventions involve providing information to physicians regarding their practices or individual patient outcomes. Two-way communication maintained over time allows for the convergence of ideas between teachers and learners—a central component of communication theory.[78] The addition of audit and feedback mechanisms and reminders can help facilitate change in practice behavior.[49,79–81] Audit and feedback techniques encompass any summary of clinical performance over a specified period and can include reminders or recommendations for clinical action.

Conditions proposed for successful feedback strategies include (1) physician recognition of need for improvement, (2) physician ability to act on information, (3) prospective reminders rather than retrospective feedback, and (4) achievable target expectations.[82–86] Examples of such systems include targeted messaging and critical incident defusing.

Targeted messaging

With e-mail systems, electronic feedback is easily accomplished within time constraints. Previous work has demonstrated the use of electronic mail-based case discussions as part of a successful multilevel intervention to improve hand-washing behavior[87] among physicians. From the perspective of addressing knowledge transformation barriers, an effective audit-feedback/reminder system addresses elements of outcome expectancy, lack of awareness and familiarity, lack of agreement, and external barriers. Combining hospital-specific data with brief reminders or tips on acute stroke care may further enhance recall of the message. This method also allows incorporation of pertinent new stroke literature, highlighting of local stroke treatment successes, distribution of printable reminders regarding tPA use in stroke, and promotion of access to other electronically available stroke treatment tools (triage and personal device assistant stroke protocols).

Critical incident defusing

Health care professionals are regularly featured in the literature exploring critical incident stress and the results of such critical incidents may include a sudden change in the daily standard operating procedures for those experiencing them. It is easy to conceive that the occurrence of an intracerebral hemorrhage, even after appropriate use of tPA in stroke, could alter future willingness to consider acute stroke treatment. Given that a small percentage of patients experience such events, a plan to address such events should be considered.

Critical incident defusing is an abbreviated form of critical incident stress debriefing, typically lasts less than 1 hour, and is designed to resolve the emotional content of an incident.[88] The critical incident defusing target should involve the treating physician, consultants, and staff. The session should be conducted by respected, trained colleagues and based on the three components of the critical incident defusing process: introduction, exploration, and information.

The objective is to provide professional support in a review of the process leading to the treatment decision. This review should be conducted in a descriptive manner and avoid performance critique.

Champion Development

Although guidelines and education by themselves may not change practice, evidence exists that providing them to local opinion leaders seems to hold substantial promise in altering physician behavior and maintaining the change. These educational influentials are opinion leaders within a community who influence the acceptance of an innovation or practice by that community.[89]

Interventions that target these people may be effective in altering local consensus or agreement regarding a guideline or treatment process.[90,91] In one study, cesarean delivery rates fell dramatically after opinion leaders were recruited and trained to promote compliance with a guideline for the management of women who had a previous cesarean section.[92] In another study, significant changes in antibiotic use were found when authoritative senior staff members were targeted for person-to-person messaging on appropriate use in conjunction with ordering reminders.[93]

To increase the likelihood that emergency physicians will adhere to recommendations for tPA use in stroke such opinion leaders should be identified and encouraged to champion stroke care. Searches for such leaders need not be restricted to within the emergency department itself. Local neurologists, internists, hospitalists, and vascular specialists may also serve in this role.

Academic Detailing

Although targeting only local opinion leaders is an efficient strategy to alter physician behavior, the process known as academic detailing—targeting populations of individual physicians for individual contact—has proved remarkably effective in almost every study in which it has been used.[94–97] Limitations of targeting individual physicians include the time and expense of contacting each physician; however, departmental staff meetings may allow efficient access to entire hospital populations of specific physicians.

Administrative Intervention

Administrative interventions can effect behavior change by creating or removing barriers to alter practice (eg, enhancing CT access for stroke, providing stroke treatment protocols, providing thrombolytic stroke expert access, and so forth). In the area of changing physician prescribing habits, administrative interventions have proved extremely successful in reducing drug costs by altering available selections or requiring drug selection review.[98] An easily recognizable national administrative intervention has been the monitoring of the time for early antibiotic delivery in emergency patients who have pneumonia.

As Greco and Eisenberg[46] note, however, there is a risk in achieving desired changes in physician practice that may ultimately cause patient harm. They cite a Medicaid program limiting reimbursement for prescription drugs that successfully reduced the number of drugs prescribed, but inadvertently increased the rate of admission to nursing homes.[99] Caution is thus advised in implementing administrative interventions because important events may go unrecognized if there is no evaluation of their impact.

POTENTIAL IMPACT OF KNOWLEDGE TRANSLATION SUCCESS IN STROKE

Recent work in other fields has demonstrated the dramatic impact successful knowledge translation can have in improving health care. In 2006, Provonost and colleagues[100] reported that an evidence-based intervention resulted in a large and sustained reduction (up to 66%) in rates of catheter-related bloodstream infection. Their intervention incorporated local champion development and training, audit/feedback mechanisms, education, and protocols (checklists) to ensure adherence to infection-control practices in 108 ICUs.

With respect to stroke and emergency medicine, previous studies have demonstrated community and academic hospitals can deliver tPA effectively.[4,37,59,60,101–105] Numerous barriers exist to expanding the delivery of tPA, however.[31,106] Only limited data currently exist on proven methods to overcome these barriers and increase physician and hospital use of tPA. One study, using a quasi-experimental design, evaluated a combination of community and professional education to increase thrombolytic use in stroke in emergency departments in rural east Texas. Treatments increased from a preintervention rate of 2.2% to a postintervention rate of 11.3% ($P = .007$), with the data suggesting the professional education component was the critical element in increasing use.[1,10] The change seemed durable; however, the study was limited by its single community setting.[1]

Currently, a cluster-randomization, multicenter, controlled trial evaluating a standardized, multilevel barrier assessment and educational intervention to increase tPA use in community hospitals and their associated emergency departments is underway, with completion anticipated in 2010 (the INSTINCT Trial, NIH R01 NS50372). The intervention under assessment incorporates many of the above elements in its design.

Assuming 500,000 ischemic strokes per year in the United States,[107] an efficient educational/behavior change process that could generate a modest 4% increase in appropriate tPA delivery could translate to an additional 20,000 treated patients per year. This practice potentially returns a minimum of 2200 stroke victims (11%) to the community normal—with added improvement across the entire spectrum of neurologic outcomes for patients who do not achieve normal status.[20]

REFERENCES

1. Morgenstern LB, Staub L, Chan W, et al. Improving delivery of acute stroke therapy: the TLL temple foundation stroke project. Stroke 2002;33(1):160–6.
2. Chiu D KD, Villar-Cordova C, Kasner SE, et al. Intravenous tissue plasminogen activator for acute ischemic stroke: feasibility, safety, and efficacy in the first year of clinical practice. Stroke 1998;29(1):18–22.
3. Katzan IL, Furlan AJ, Lloyd LE, et al. Use of tissue-type plasminogen activator for acute ischemic stroke: the Cleveland area experience. JAMA 2000;283(9):1151–8.
4. Chapman KM, Woolfenden AR, Graeb D, et al. Intravenous tissue plasminogen activator for acute ischemic stroke: a Canadian hospital's experience. Stroke 2000;31(12):2920–4.
5. Reed SD, Cramer SC, Blough DK, et al. Treatment with tissue plasminogen activator and inpatient mortality rates for patients with ischemic stroke treated in community hospitals. Stroke 2001;32(8):1832–40.
6. Reeves MJ, Arora S, Broderick JP, et al. Acute stroke care in the US: results from 4 pilot prototypes of the Paul Coverdell national acute stroke registry. Stroke 2005;36(6):1232–40.
7. Schumacher HC, Bateman BT, Boden-Albala B, et al. Use of thrombolysis in acute ischemic stroke: analysis of the nationwide inpatient sample 1999 to 2004. Ann Emerg Med 2007;50(2):99–107.
8. Kleindorfer D, Kissela B, Schneider A, et al. Eligibility for recombinant tissue plasminogen activator in acute ischemic stroke: a population-based study. Stroke 2004;35(2):e27–9.
9. Grotta JC, Burgin WS, El-Mitwalli A, et al. Intravenous tissue-type plasminogen activator therapy for ischemic stroke: Houston experience 1996 to 2000. Arch Neurol 2001;58(12):2009–13.
10. Morgenstern LB, Bartholomew LK, Grotta JC, et al. Sustained benefit of a community and professional intervention to increase acute stroke therapy. Arch Intern Med 2003;163(18):2198–202.
11. Lyden P, Hickenbottom S. Professional education task force report. In: Improving the chain of recovery for acute stroke in your community; 2003. National Institute of Neurologic Disorders and Stroke, Publication #NIH 03-5348.
12. Canadian Institute of Health Research. Knowledge translation strategy 2004–2009: innovation in action. Available at: http://www.cihr-irsc.gc.ca/e/26574.html. Accessed April 29, 2008.

13. Sung NS, Crowley WF Jr, Genel M, et al. Central challenges facing the national clinical research enterprise. JAMA 2003;289(10):1278–87.
14. Lang ES, Wyer PC, Haynes RB. Knowledge translation: closing the evidence-to-practice gap. Ann Emerg Med 2007;49(3):355–63.
15. Lang ES, Wyer PC, Eskin B. Executive summary: knowledge translation in emergency medicine: establishing a research agenda and guide map for evidence uptake. Acad Emerg Med 2007;14(11):915–8.
16. Joos S, Hickam D. How health professionals influence health behavior: patient provider interaction and health care outcomes. In: Glanz K, Lewis F, Rimer B, editors. Health behavior and health education: theory, research and practice. San Francisco (CA): Jossey Bass; 1990. p. 216–41.
17. Hickenbottom S, Morgenstern L. Educating North America: lessons learned. Seminars in Cerebrovascular Disease and Stroke 2001;1(2):167–75.
18. Sutton S. Social-psychological approaches to understanding addictive behaviours: attitude-behaviour and decision-making models. Br J Addict 1987;82(4):355–70.
19. Weinstein N. Testing four competing theories of health-protective behavior. Health Psychol 1993;12(4):324–33.
20. Anonymous. Tissue plasminogen activator for acute ischemic stroke. The National Institute of Neurological Disorders and Stroke rt-PA stroke study group. [see comments]. N Engl J Med 1995;333(24):1581–7.
21. Kwiatkowski TG, Libman RB, Frankel M, et al. Effects of tissue plasminogen activator for acute ischemic stroke at one year. National Institute of Neurological Disorders and Stroke recombinant tissue plasminogen activator stroke study group. [see comments]. N Engl J Med 1999;340(23):1781–7.
22. Anonymous. Randomised controlled trial of streptokinase, aspirin, and combination of both in treatment of acute ischaemic stroke. Multicentre acute stroke trial—Italy (MAST-I) group. [comment] [see comments]. Lancet 1995;346(8989):1509–14.
23. Anonymous. Thrombolytic therapy with streptokinase in acute ischemic stroke. The multicenter acute stroke trial—Europe study group. [see comments]. N Engl J Med 1996;335(3):145–50.
24. Clark WM, Wissman S, Albers GW, et al. Recombinant tissue-type plasminogen activator (alteplase) for ischemic stroke 3 to 5 hours after symptom onset. The ATLANTIS study: a randomized controlled trial. Alteplase thrombolysis for acute noninterventional therapy in ischemic stroke. [see comments]. JAMA 1999;282(21):2019–26.
25. Donnan GA, Davis SM, Chambers BR, et al. Streptokinase for acute ischemic stroke with relationship to time of administration: Australian streptokinase (ASK) trial study group. JAMA 1996;276(12):961–6.
26. Hacke W, Kaste M, Fieschi C, et al. Intravenous thrombolysis with recombinant tissue plasminogen activator for acute hemispheric stroke. The European cooperative acute stroke study (ECASS). [see comments]. JAMA 1995;274(13):1017–25.
27. Hacke W, Kaste M, Fieschi C, et al. Randomised double-blind placebo-controlled trial of thrombolytic therapy with intravenous alteplase in acute ischaemic stroke (ECASS II). Second European-Australasian acute stroke study investigators. [see comments]. Lancet 1998;352(9136):1245–51.
28. Wahlgren N, Ahmed N, Davalos A, et al. Thrombolysis with alteplase for acute ischaemic stroke in the safe implementation of thrombolysis in stroke-monitoring study (SITS-MOST): an observational study. Lancet 2007;369(9558):275–82.

29. Anonymous. Practice advisory: thrombolytic therapy for acute ischemic stroke— summary statement. Report of the quality standards subcommittee of the American Academy of Neurology. Neurology 1996;47(3):835–9.

30. Adams HP Jr, del Zoppo G, Alberts MJ, et al. Guidelines for the early management of adults with ischemic stroke: a guideline from the American Heart Association/American Stroke Association stroke council, clinical cardiology council, cardiovascular radiology and intervention council, and the atherosclerotic peripheral vascular disease and quality of care outcomes in research interdisciplinary working groups: the American Academy of Neurology affirms the value of this guideline as an educational tool for neurologists. Stroke 2007;38(5): 1655–711.

31. Anonymous. Proceedings of a National Symposium on rapid identification and treatment of acute stroke. In: John R, Marler PWJ, Marian Emr, editors. Rapid identification and treatment of acute stroke; 1997; Bethesda (MD): National Institute of Neurological Disorders and Stroke; 1997.

32. Improving the chain of recovery for acute stroke in your community; 2003. National Institute of Neurological Disorders and Stroke, Publication #NIH 03-5348.

33. ACEP agrees with reservations to new stroke guidelines. ACEP News. October 1996;3.

34. ACEP Policy Statement: Use of intravenous tPA for the management of acute stroke in the emergency department. American College of Emergency Physicians, 2002. Available at: http://www.acep.org/practres.aspx?id=29834. Accessed November, 2002.

35. AAEM Work Group on Thrombolytic Therapy in Stroke. Position statement of the American Academy of Emergency Medicine on the use of intravenous thrombolytic therapy in the treatment of stroke. Available at: http://www.aaem.org/positionstatements/thrombolytictherapy.php. Accessed on June 2008.

36. Ingall TJ, O'Fallon WM, Asplund K, et al. Findings from the reanalysis of the NINDS tissue plasminogen activator for acute ischemic stroke treatment trial. Stroke 2004;35(10):2418–24.

37. Albers GW, Bates VE, Clark WM, et al. Intravenous tissue-type plasminogen activator for treatment of acute stroke: the standard treatment with alteplase to reverse stroke (STARS) study. [see comments]. JAMA 2000;283(9): 1145–50.

38. Hill MD, Buchan AM. Thrombolysis for acute ischemic stroke: results of the Canadian alteplase for stroke effectiveness study. CMAJ 2005;172(10):1307–12.

39. Kwan J, Hand P, Sandercock P. A systematic review of barriers to delivery of thrombolysis for acute stroke. Age Ageing 2004;33(2):116–21.

40. Rogers W, Bowlby L, Chandra N, et al. Treatment of myocardial infarction in the United States (1990 to 1993). Observations from the National Registry of Myocardial Infarction. Circulation 1994;90(4):2103–14.

41. Kunnel B, Heller M. Thrombolytics and stroke: what do emergency medicine residents perceive? Acad Emerg Med 1999;6(11):1174–6.

42. Brown DL, Barsan WG, Lisabeth LD, et al. Survey of emergency physicians about recombinant tissue plasminogen activator for acute ischemic stroke. Ann Emerg Med 2005;46(1):56–60.

43. Cabana MD, Rand CS, Powe NR, et al. Why don't physicians follow clinical practice guidelines? A framework for improvement. JAMA 1999;282(15):1458–65.

44. Cabana MD, Ebel BE, Cooper-Patrick L, et al. Barriers pediatricians face when using asthma practice guidelines. Arch Pediatr Adolesc Med 2000;154(7): 685–93.

45. Meurer WJ, Frederiksen SM, Majersik JJ, et al. Qualitative data collection and analysis methods: the INSTINCT trial. Acad Emerg Med 2007;14(11):1064–71.
46. Greco PJ, Eisenberg JM. Changing physicians' practices. N Engl J Med 1993; 329(17):1271–3.
47. Browner W, Baron R, Solkowitz S, et al. Physician management of hypercholesterolemia. A randomized trial of continuing medical education. West J Med 1994; 161(6):572–8.
48. Boissel J, Collet J, Alborini A, et al. Education program for general practitioners on breast and cervical cancer screening: a randomized trial. PRE.SA.GF collaborative group. Rev Epidemiol Sante Publique 1995;43(6):541–7.
49. Davis D, O'Brien MAT, Freemantle N, et al. Impact of formal continuing medical education: do conferences, workshops, rounds, and other traditional continuing education activities change physician behavior or health care outcomes? JAMA 1999;282(9):867–74.
50. Kottke TE, Brekke ML, Solberg LI, et al. A randomized trial to increase smoking intervention by physicians. Doctors helping smokers, round I. JAMA 1989; 261(14):2101–6.
51. Levinson W, Roter D. The effects of two continuing medical education programs on communication skills of practicing primary care physicians. J Gen Intern Med 1993;8(6):318–24.
52. Maiman LA, Becker MH, Liptak GS, et al. Improving pediatricians' compliance-enhancing practices. A randomized trial. Am J Dis Child 1988;142(7):773–9.
53. Ockene IS, Hebert JR, Ockene JK, et al. Effect of training and a structured office practice on physician-delivered nutrition counseling: the Worcester-area trial for counseling in hyperlipidemia (WATCH). Am J Prev Med 1996;12(4):252–8.
54. Roter DL, Hall JA, Kern DE, et al. Improving physicians' interviewing skills and reducing patients' emotional distress. A randomized clinical trial. Arch Intern Med 1995;155(17):1877–84.
55. White CW, Albanese MA, Brown DD, et al. The effectiveness of continuing medical education in changing the behavior of physicians caring for patients with acute myocardial infarction. A controlled randomized trial. Ann Intern Med 1985;102(5):686–92.
56. IV t-PA Interventional therapy for acute stroke patients: a debate. Canadian Association of Emergency Physicians Annual Scientific Meeting. Calgary, Alberta, Canada, 2002.
57. Hoffman JR. Predicted impact of intravenous thrombolysis. Another trial is needed. BMJ 2000;320(7240):1007.
58. Hoffman JR. Alteplase for stroke. Why were these authors of the commentaries chosen? BMJ 2002;324(7353):1581 [author reply].
59. Smith RW, Scott PA, Grant RJ, et al. Emergency physician treatment of acute stroke with recombinant tissue plasminogen activator: a retrospective analysis. Academic Emergency Medicine 1999;6(6):618–25.
60. Scott P, Davis L, Frederiksen S, et al. Emergency physician administration of rt-PA in acute stroke: five-year analysis of treatment and outcome. [abstract]. Acad Emerg Med 2002;9(5):447.
61. Scott P, Smith R, Davis L, et al. Time analysis of emergency physician delivery of rt-PA in acute ischemic stroke. [abstract A327]. Acad Emerg Med 2000;7(5): 535.
62. Scott PA, Smith RW, Chudnofsky CR, et al. Emergency physician administration of rt-PA in acute stroke: analysis of treatment and outcome. [abstract]. Stroke 1999;30(1):244.

63. Scott P, Silbergleit R. Misdiagnosis of stroke in tissue plasminogen activator-treated patients: characteristics and outcomes. Ann Emerg Med 2003;42(5):611–8.

64. Scott P, Silbergleit R, Frederiksen S, et al. Long term mortality in stroke patients treated with TPA: emergency physicians vs NINDS. [abstract]. Acad Emerg Med 2003;10(5):433.

65. Bandura A. Social foundations of thought and action: a social cognitive theory. Engelwood Cliffs (NJ): Prentice-Hall, Inc.; 1986.

66. Hayward RS. Clinical practice guidelines on trial. CMAJ 1997;156(12):1725–7.

67. Lomas J, Anderson GM, Domnick-Pierre K, et al. Do practice guidelines guide practice? The effect of a consensus statement on the practice of physicians. N Engl J Med 1989;321(19):1306–11.

68. Woolf SH. Practice guidelines: a new reality in medicine. III. Impact on patient care. Arch Intern Med 1993;153(23):2646–55.

69. Gass DA, Curry L. Physicians' and nurses' retention of knowledge and skill after training in cardiopulmonary resuscitation. Can Med Assoc J 1983;128(5):550–1.

70. Lum ME, Galletly DC. Resuscitation skills of first year postgraduate doctors. N Z Med J 1989;102(873):406–8.

71. Cappelle C, Paul RI. Educating residents: the effects of a mock code program. Resuscitation 1996;31(2):107–11.

72. Funkhouser MJ, Hayward MF. Multidisciplinary mock codes: dream it, plan it, do it, rate it. J Nurses Staff Dev 1989;5(5):231–7.

73. Main DS, Cohen SJ, DiClemente CC. Measuring physician readiness to change cancer screening: preliminary results. Am J Prev Med 1995;11(1):54–8.

74. Frey JL, Jahnke HK, Goslar PW, et al. tPA by telephone: extending the benefits of a comprehensive stroke center. Neurology 2005;64(1):154–6.

75. Vaishnav AG, Pettigrew LC, Ryan S. Telephonic guidance of systemic thrombolysis in acute ischemic stroke: safety outcome in rural hospitals. Clin Neurol Neurosurg 2008.

76. Schwab S, Vatankhah B, Kukla C, et al. Long-term outcome after thrombolysis in telemedical stroke care. Neurology 2007;69(9):898–903.

77. Schwamm LH, Rosenthal ES, Hirshberg A, et al. Virtual teleStroke support for the emergency department evaluation of acute stroke. Acad Emerg Med 2004; 11(11):1193–7.

78. Berlo D. The process of communication: an introduction to theory and practice. New York: Holt, Rinehart & Winston; 1960.

79. Davis DA, Thomson MA, Oxman AD, et al. Changing physician performance. A systematic review of the effect of continuing medical education strategies. JAMA 1995;274(9):700–5.

80. Davis DA, Taylor-Vaisey A. Translating guidelines into practice. A systematic review of theoretic concepts, practical experience and research evidence in the adoption of clinical practice guidelines. CMAJ 1997;157(4):408–16.

81. Mazmanian PE, Davis DA. Continuing medical education and the physician as a learner: guide to the evidence. JAMA 2002;288(9):1057–60.

82. Pimlott NJ, Hux JE, Wilson LM, et al. Educating physicians to reduce benzodiazepine use by elderly patients: a randomized controlled trial. CMAJ 2003; 168(7):835–9.

83. Parrino TA. The nonvalue of retrospective peer comparison feedback in containing hospital antibiotic costs. Am J Med 1989;86(4):442–8.

84. Hershey CO, Goldberg HI, Cohen DI. The effect of computerized feedback coupled with a newsletter upon outpatient prescribing charges. A randomized controlled trial. Med Care 1988;26(1):88–94.

85. McPhee SJ, Bird JA, Jenkins CN, et al. Promoting cancer screening. A randomized, controlled trial of three interventions. Arch Intern Med 1989;149(8):1866–72.

86. Tierney WM, Hui SL, McDonald CJ. Delayed feedback of physician performance versus immediate reminders to perform preventive care. Effects on physician compliance. Med Care 1986;24(8):659–66.

87. Salemi C, Canola MT, Eck EK. Hand washing and physicians: how to get them together. Infect Control Hosp Epidemiol 2002;23(1):32–5.

88. Oster NS, Doyle CJ. Critical incident stress and challenges for the emergency workplace. Emerg Med Clin North Am 2000;18(2):339–53, x–xi.

89. Greer AL. The state of the art versus the state of the science. The diffusion of new medical technologies into practice. Int J Technol Assess Health Care 1988;4(1):5–26.

90. Mittman BS, Tonesk X, Jacobson PD. Implementing clinical practice guidelines: social influence strategies and practitioner behavior change. QRB Qual Rev Bull 1992;18(12):413–22.

91. Soumerai SB, McLaughlin TJ, Gurwitz JH, et al. Effect of local medical opinion leaders on quality of care for acute myocardial infarction: a randomized controlled trial. JAMA 1998;279(17):1358–63.

92. Lomas J, Enkin M, Anderson GM, et al. Opinion leaders vs audit and feedback to implement practice guidelines. Delivery after previous cesarean section. JAMA 1991;265(17):2202–7.

93. Everitt DE, Soumerai SB, Avorn J, et al. Changing surgical antimicrobial prophylaxis practices through education targeted at senior department leaders. Infect Control Hosp Epidemiol 1990;11(11):578–83.

94. Soumerai SB, Salem-Schatz S, Avorn J, et al. A controlled trial of educational outreach to improve blood transfusion practice. JAMA 1993;270(8):961–6.

95. Avorn J, Soumerai SB. A new approach to reducing suboptimal drug use. JAMA 1983;250(13):1752–3.

96. Ray WA, Schaffner W, Federspiel CF. Persistence of improvement in antibiotic prescribing in office practice. JAMA 1985;253(12):1774–6.

97. Ray WA, Blazer DG 2nd, Schaffner W, et al. Reducing long-term diazepam prescribing in office practice. A controlled trial of educational visits. JAMA 1986;256(18):2536–9.

98. Coleman RW, Rodondi LC, Kaubisch S, et al. Cost-effectiveness of prospective and continuous parenteral antibiotic control: experience at the Palo Alto Veterans Affairs Medical Center from 1987 to 1989. Am J Med 1991;90(4):439–44.

99. Soumerai SB, Ross-Degnan D, Avorn J, et al. Effects of medicaid drug-payment limits on admission to hospitals and nursing homes. N Engl J Med 1991;325(15):1072–7.

100. Pronovost P, Needham D, Berenholtz S, et al. An intervention to decrease catheter-related bloodstream infections in the ICU. N Engl J Med 2006;355(26):2725–32.

101. Davenport J, Hanson SK, Altafullah IM, et al. tPA: a rural network experience. Stroke 2000;31(6):1457–8.

102. Grond M, Stenzel C, Schmulling S, et al. Early intravenous thrombolysis for acute ischemic stroke in a community-based approach. Stroke 1998;29(8):1544–9.

103. Katzan IL, Sila CA, Furlan AJ. Community use of intravenous tissue plasminogen activator for acute stroke: results of the brain matters stroke management survey. Stroke 2001;32(4):861–5.

104. Wang DZ, Rose JA, Honings DS, et al. Treating acute stroke patients with intravenous tPA. The OSF stroke network experience. Stroke 2000;31(1):77–81.
105. Tanne D, Bates VE, Verro P, et al. Initial clinical experience with IV tissue plasminogen activator for acute ischemic stroke: a multicenter survey. The t-PA stroke survey group. Neurology 1999;53(2):424–7.
106. Alberts MJ. tPA in acute ischemic stroke: United States experience and issues for the future. Neurology 1998;51(3 Suppl 3):S53–5.
107. Broderick J, Brott T, Kothari R, et al. The Greater Cincinnati/Northern Kentucky stroke study: preliminary first-ever and total incidence rates of stroke among blacks. Stroke 1998;29(2):415–21.

Therapeutic Hypothermia for Neuroprotection

C. Jessica Dine, MD[a], Benjamin S. Abella, MD, MPhil[b],*

KEYWORDS

• Cardiac arrest • Hypothermia • Resuscitation

Therapeutic hypothermia (TH) represents the intentional induction of a lowered core body temperature.[1] One of the first case series describing the clinical application of hypothermia was published in 1945,[2] which led to the notion of hypothermia for intracerebral aneurysm surgery and cerebral protection during circulatory arrest to allow for intracardiac operations in a bloodless field.[3–6] Over the last several decades, TH has been employed during cardiac surgery using cardiopulmonary bypass or during neurosurgical procedures in the hope of protecting the brain from ischemic injury.[7] More recently, it has become a management step in providing victims of sudden cardiac arrest (SCA) the best chance of survival with a good neurologic recovery. This review briefly discusses the history of induced hypothermia before focusing on resuscitative or postarrest hypothermia, the data that support it, and the practical issues pertaining to TH implementation.

BRIEF HISTORY OF THERAPEUTIC HYPOTHERMIA

Protective or pretreatment hypothermia[8] has been used since the 1950s[9] for cerebral protection by extending tolerance to anoxia during cardiovascular surgery;[4] however, the concept of TH dates as far back as the ancient Greeks. In fact, Hippocrates advocated treating bleeding patients by packing them in snow and ice.[10] Baron Larrey, Napoleon's chief battlefield surgeon, observed that injured soldiers who were left in the cold had a better survival rate than soldiers who were rewarmed.[11] Since then TH has been investigated in the treatment of many different illnesses, including myocardial infarction, stroke, and sepsis.[9,12,13] Early animal models using hypothermia for cardiac arrest resuscitation suggested mixed results.[14] Although other clinical data on TH appeared promising,[15,16] postarrest hypothermia was

[a] Division of Pulmonary, Allergy and Critical Care, University of Pennsylvania, 3400 Spruce Street, Ground Ravdin, Philadelphia, PA 19104, USA
[b] Department of Emergency Medicine and Center for Resuscitation Science, University of Pennsylvania, 3400 Spruce Street, Ground Ravdin, Philadelphia, PA 19104, USA
* Corresponding author.
E-mail address: benjamin.abella@uphs.upenn.edu (B.S. Abella).

Emerg Med Clin N Am 27 (2009) 137–149
doi:10.1016/j.emc.2008.07.003
0733-8627/08/$ – see front matter © 2009 Elsevier Inc. All rights reserved.

emed.theclinics.com

abandoned until the 1980s when improved animal models to study cardiac arrest and TH were developed. Gisvold and colleagues[17] tested a multifaceted approach to resuscitation after global ischemia in a primate model that included hypothermia for 6 hours. In 1990, Leonov and colleagues[18] reported the effects of inducing hypothermia during canine cardiac arrest. In both studies, the animals whose treatment included TH showed evidence of improved neurologic outcomes.

CONTEMPORARY CLINICAL TRIALS OF POSTARREST HYPOTHERMIA

Encouraged by promising laboratory data supporting the use of TH after cardiac arrest resuscitation, several small clinical trials in the 1980s and 1990s were conducted and reported improved clinical outcomes with TH when compared with historical controls. This line of investigation culminated in three randomized controlled clinical trials of TH published in 2001–2002.[19–21] These two studies evaluated the potential impact of TH on the functional outcomes and survival rates following out-of-hospital SCA.

Bernard and colleagues[19] randomized 77 subjects after resuscitation from ventricular fibrillation (VF) cardiac arrest to receive conventional treatment under normothermic conditions or with hypothermia to a core body temperature of 33°C within several hours after the return of spontaneous circulation (ROSC). In the hypothermia group, this temperature was maintained for 12 hours. In the group treated with TH, 49% of subjects survived to be discharged to home or to a rehabilitation facility compared with 26% of subjects treated with normothermia (odds ratio, 5.25; 95% CI, 1.47–18.76).

The Hypothermia After Cardiac Arrest (HACA) study group[20] randomized 275 victims of out-of-hospital VF cardiac arrest to receive either normothermic treatment or TH with a target temperature of 32°C to 34°C over 24 hours. The neurologic outcome within 6 months was described using the Pittsburgh Cerebral Performance Category rating scale. A favorable outcome was defined as a score of 1 (good recovery) or 2 (moderate disability) on a five-item scale in which the other categories were 3 (severe disability), 4 (vegetative state), and 5 (death). The TH group demonstrated a significant improvement in functional outcome of 55% compared with 39% in the normothermia group (risk ratio, 1.40; 95% CI, 1.08–1.81). **Table 1** presents a summary of TH randomized controlled trials.

The inclusion criteria for both of these trials were fairly strict. For example, both studies included only patients who had experienced witnessed arrests with a short time interval from collapse to the initiation of cardiopulmonary resuscitation. Furthermore, the initial rhythm in all of these patients was VF or ventricular tachycardia (VT).

Table 1
Summary data from three randomized controlled trials of TH after cardiac arrest

Trial	Hypothermia (%)	Normothermia (%)	RR (95% CI)	P value
Alive at hospital discharge with favorable neurologic recovery				
HACA[20]	72/136 (55)	50/137 (39)	1.40 (1.08–1.81)	0.009
Bernard[19]	21/43 (49)	9/34 (26)	5.25 (1.47–18.76)	0.011
Hachimi-Idrissi[21]	3/16 (19)	1/14 (6)	4.25 (0.70–53.83)	0.16
Alive at 6 months with favorable neurologic recovery				
HACA	71/136 (52)	50/137 (41)	1.44 (1.11–1.76)	0.009

Abbreviations: HACA, Hypothermia After Cardiac Arrest study group; RR, relative risk.

Patients with persistent hypotension and hypoxia were also excluded; therefore, it is less clear if TH would provide similar benefits for patients with other rhythms or those that remain unstable after ROSC. Because cardiac arrest leads to myocardial and cerebral ischemia regardless of initial rhythm, it is possible that hypothermia could have a protective effect in a similar manner in these patients as well.

MECHANISMS OF HYPOTHERMIC PROTECTION

The exact mechanisms by which TH protects against cellular and tissue injury remain unclear. It is likely that multiple mechanisms are involved,[22,23] including modulation of intracellular signaling, gene expression controlling the interrelated cascades of oxidative injury, inflammation, and programmed cell death, all of which are apparently modified by cooling. Hypothermia is associated with attenuation of intermediate stages of each of these pathways after cerebral ischemia and reperfusion. Furthermore, the induction of hypothermia ultimately reduces the number of neurons lost both immediately following global cerebral ischemia[24–27] and from delayed programmed cell death.[28] In another study involving a rat liver ischemia-reperfusion model, reactive oxygen species production was diminished by maintaining the liver tissue at 34°C after reperfusion.[29] Such observations in animal models suggest that induced hypothermia can alter the effects of ischemia during and following an anoxic event such as SCA.

INTRA- VERSUS POSTARREST HYPOTHERMIA

The multiple mechanisms of cerebral injury during periods of ischemia suggest that a variety of hypothermia strategies could provide benefit and improve neurologic outcomes post cardiac arrest. Markarian and colleagues[30] aimed to elucidate the therapeutic window of TH in a rat model of focal cerebral ischemia and found that the greatest benefit was seen when it was implemented immediately following the onset of ischemia; however, in the clinical setting of SCA, the institution of intra-arrest TH may not be feasible. It is most practical to focus on implementing induced hypothermia as soon as possible following resuscitation from cardiac arrest; however, even in this more established model of hypothermia application, several specific parameters require additional discussion and further research (**Fig. 1**).

DEPTH OF HYPOTHERMIA

The depth of hypothermia is generally grouped into the categories of mild (33–36°C), moderate (28–33°C), and deep (<28°C). Although the optimal therapeutic temperature is unknown, most animal and human TH studies have employed mild-to-moderate hypothermia. Animal models have shown that moderate hypothermia provides more neuroprotection than mild hypothermia;[31–33] however, it is unknown whether such an effect would be found with deep hypothermia as well. In fact, some animal models suggest that mild hypothermia after the return of circulation provokes fewer adverse effects than colder temperatures.[34,35] Further human studies are needed to elucidate the goal core temperature to maximize the chance of complete neurologic recovery following cardiac arrest. Based on the recent clinical trials by Bernard and colleagues[19] and the HACA study group,[20] current recommendations state that patients sustaining out-of-hospital cardiac arrest should receive mild TH with temperatures of 32°C to 34°C.[36]

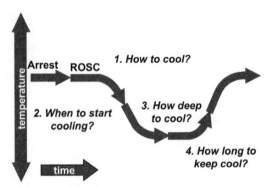

Fig. 1. Four fundamental parameters of TH that remain active areas of research.

TIMING AND DURATION OF HYPOTHERMIA

Animal data generally show that immediate TH is superior to delayed hypothermia,[37] suggesting that the earlier cooling is initiated after reperfusion following a cardiac arrest, the better the potential for a favorable neurologic outcome. Nevertheless, clinical studies demonstrate a significant therapeutic effect even when cooling is delayed by several hours after ROSC;[19,20,38] therefore, the importance of rapidity of cooling remains controversial, with some investigators arguing that the response to cooling may not actually be time sensitive, at least within a several hour time window.[39] Pending further investigation of this controversy, it is generally agreed that TH should be initiated as soon as possible. TH should be initiated at any point within several hours of resuscitation if it was not started immediately after ROSC.

Similarly, the most effective duration of TH is unknown and has ranged from 6 to 48 hours following SCA. Bernard and colleagues[19] induced moderate hypothermia (33°C) and maintained this temperature for 12 hours. The HACA group maintained their target temperature of 32°C to 34°C for 24 hours.[20] Although the exact duration of induced hypothermia following cardiac arrest is unknown, recommendations suggest a time course of 12 to 24 hours based on these trials.[36]

COOLING METHODS

A recent survey of German critical care physicians[40] investigated the methods employed in their ICUs and revealed that most centers used external cooling in the form of cold packs (82%) with or without cold intravenous saline infusions (80%) for hypothermia induction. Many clinical studies have also used external cooling systems, including cooling blankets,[41] direct contact with cold water or ice,[42] or an external cooling helmet.[21] Although these methods are relatively effective in inducing mild hypothermia, they may be limited by the human protective mechanisms against hypothermia. These mechanisms include the ability of humans to generate thermal energy to defend against cooling through shivering, the ability to redirect blood flow away from extremities or skin to prevent heat loss, and the low mass-to-surface area ratio of the human body. Furthermore, most external cooling methods do not automatically maintain the body temperature within the desired range, and unintentional overcooling is common using ice packs and conventional cooling blankets. One study found that in 32 cases in which external cooling methods were used to induce mild TH, 63% of the patients were overcooled, increasing the risk for adverse effects.[43]

These limitations have led to the development of novel cooling techniques, including peritoneal cooling,[44] catheters with closed cooling systems,[45] and pulmonary cooling[46,47] in animal models. Clinical trials are necessary to assess whether these techniques are feasible for TH in humans.

Noninvasive external cooling devices that use thermoregulatory control units coupled to thermometers to precisely maintain a given target body temperature have recently been studied.[48] These systems circulate cold fluids through external pads or wraps which are applied to the patient's skin. In addition, these devices can automatically change the temperature of the circulating water in response to the preset target temperature and actual measured patient temperature.

Endovascular cooling represents another technique that allows for rapid induction and careful maintenance of reduced temperatures; therefore, it is preferred at many institutions. This method involves the insertion of a closed-loop, coolant-filled catheter in the vena cava. The blood is cooled as it circulates past the inserted catheter.[49] One clinical study compared the use of endovascular cooling with the application of ice packs for 24 hours among resuscitated patients sustaining SCA.[50] The group cooled with an endovascular device reached a lower mean core temperature of 32.9°C compared with 36.1°C in the group cooled with ice packs.

Further investigations into which methods of cooling are most effective for rapid induction and maintenance are required in the near future. Additionally, newer technologies being developed in the animal laboratory will likely provide additional opportunities in the clinical domain.

PARALYSIS

Shivering as a natural defense mechanism against hypothermia generates heat that may impede the process of inducing or maintaining TH. Shivering in the process of heat generation also increases metabolic rates, a process that may worsen cellular injury. During the induction of TH, shivering is likely to occur when the core temperature reaches 34°C to 36°C but then diminishes when the temperature falls below 34°C;[51] therefore, it may be possible to either initiate paralysis only during cooling and rewarming or to induce paralysis throughout the induction and maintenance of hypothermia. In the studies by Bernard and colleagues and the HACA group, paralysis was induced using neuromuscular blocking agents to prevent shivering.[19,20] In the HACA study pancuronium was given for 36 hours,[20] whereas in the study by Bernard and colleagues[19] vecuronium was used only as needed to treat clinically apparent shivering. The immediate adverse effects of paralytics include the masking of seizures that may be induced by TH [52] and hypotension;[53] however, if used on an as needed basis or reserved for the cooling and rewarming process only (while the core body temperature falls between 34°C and 36°C), these adverse phenomena may potentially be mitigated. Other options to control shivering may include pharmacologic agents such as meperidine, buspirone, or interventions with deep sedation.

ADVERSE EVENTS OF INDUCED HYPOTHERMIA

Although uncommon in clinical studies of mild hypothermia, hypothermia has the potential to induce coagulopathy, infection, pancreatitis, renal dysfunction, electrolyte abnormalities, and arrhythmias.[52] In the two recent randomized trials of TH, these adverse events were found to be of minimal clinical occurrence and consequence.[19,20] For example, none of the adverse events identified in the HACA trial were found to be different from that in the normothermia group.[20] In the hypothermia group, the most common side effects included bleeding (26% in the TH group versus 19% in the control group), arrhythmias (36% versus 32%), pneumonia (37% versus 29%), and renal failure (both 10%).

Coagulopathy associated with cooling can be secondary to an impaired coagulation cascade as well as TH-induced thrombocytopenia and reduced platelet function.[52] A mild thrombocytopenia is most commonly observed with rare bleeding events. Other potential side effects during cooling include insulin resistance and electrolyte abnormalities including hypokalemia, hypomagnesemia, hypophosphatemia, and hypocalcemia, largely through hypothermia-induced diuresis mechanisms. Although a rise in serum amylase is common, clinical pancreatitis is rare. Other laboratory abnormalities that may rarely occur but cause a significant clinical adverse event include mild abnormalities in liver enzymes and an increase in serum lactate levels (although this may be more related to the phenomenon of ischemia-reperfusion than TH). **Box 1** lists potential TH adverse effects.

CURRENT RECOMMENDATIONS AND GUIDELINES FOR POSTARREST HYPOTHERMIA

Both the European Resuscitation Council and the American Heart Association (AHA) have recently published guidelines for postarrest hypothermia.[36,54] The Advanced Life Support Task Force of the International Liaison Committee on Resuscitation (ILCOR) recommends that "unconscious adult patients with spontaneous circulation after out-of-hospital cardiac arrest should be cooled to 32°C to 34°C for 12 to 24 hours when the initial rhythm was VF" and that such cooling "may also be beneficial for other rhythms or in-hospital cardiac arrest."[36]

These guidelines have stressed that cooling should be initiated as soon as possible after ROSC but also suggest that it may be successful even if delayed up to 4 to

---

Box 1
Potential adverse effects from hypothermia, with more common occurrences marked with asterisks (*)

Cardiac
    Bradycardia*
    Premature ventricular contractions
    VF
Metabolic
    Hypokalemia
    Hypomagnesemia
    Hypocalcemia
    Diuresis/volume contraction*
Hematologic
    Coagulopathy*
    Thrombocytopenia
    Platelet dysfunction
Neurologic
    Shivering*
    Seizures

6 hours. Although the ILCOR recommendations point out that induced hypothermia may also be beneficial after in-hospital cardiac arrest or in patients with non-VF/VT initial rhythms, they warn against using TH in patients with "severe cardiogenic shock or life-threatening arrhythmias, pregnant patients, or patients with primary coagulopathy" until further data are available.[36]

More recently, the AHA also incorporated hypothermia recommendations into their 2005 resuscitation guideline update.[54] Similarly to the ILCOR recommendations, the AHA recommends cooling for comatose survivors of out-of-hospital VF arrest, but also mentions the possible benefit of cooling in-hospital arrest patients and patients with other arrest rhythms. In the nomenclature of the AHA guidelines, TH is now a class IIa recommendation for out-of-hospital, comatose survivors of a VF arrest, whereas TH for victims of SCA with other initial rhythms or in-hospital arrest is a class IIb recommendation.

CURRENT USE OF POSTARREST HYPOTHERMIA

The ILCOR recommendations were published in 2003. Recent investigations have demonstrated that TH is not routinely practiced at most institutions in the United States. An Internet-based survey of US physicians[55] concluded that 87% of the 265 physicians who responded had never used TH following SCA, although the majority of surveyed physicians specialized in emergency medicine (41%), critical care medicine (13%), and cardiology (24%). The most common reasons cited for nonuse included the lack of enough data, the lack of incorporation of hypothermia into advanced cardiovascular life support protocols, and the difficulty of using cooling methods.

A similar Internet-based survey was conducted among physicians in the United States, United Kingdom, and Finland.[56] The majority of physicians again reported never having used TH (ie, 74% of US and 64% of non-US physicians). The most commonly cited reasons were identical to those given in previous survey work. A survey of pediatric intensivists[57] demonstrated similarly low rates of use, with only 9% replying that they always used and 38% that they sometimes used resuscitative hypothermia. The most common reasons listed were the likelihood of patient recovery, the absence of life-limiting disease, and the presence of coma for more than 1 hour after resuscitation.

Despite compelling data supporting the use of induced hypothermia following cardiac arrest, as well as the publication of the ILCOR and AHA recommendations regarding TH, this method to improve the neurologic outcomes of SCA victims has not been widely adopted. This finding demonstrates the need for further education and training as well as practical guides for the implementation of hypothermia. Explicit hypothermia protocols may need to be included in algorithms for advanced cardiovascular life support in the future, and hypothermia methods will require standardization. Recent modeling has estimated the substantial estimated effect of widespread adoption of hypothermia for the treatment of comatose survivors of cardiac arrest.[58]

THE DEVELOPMENT OF HYPOTHERMIA PROTOCOLS

Although the low use rate of TH following SCA highlights the need for further training and education as well as the design and increased availability of established protocols, few data are available on how to design such a protocol or on the effect of such protocols on hospital use. Following the ILCOR recommendations, the European Resuscitation Council Hypothermia After Cardiac Arrest Registry was founded to monitor the implementation of TH, to observe the feasibility of adherence to guidelines, and to document the effects of hypothermic treatment in terms of complications and outcome.[59] During a 2-year period, 650 patients who had a cardiac arrest with ROSC were entered into the registry. Of these patients, 79% received TH via different methods, including the use of an endovascular device, ice packs, cooling blankets, and cold fluids. Although this study demonstrates that the implementation of TH is feasible, it also illustrates that no standardized protocol has been uniformly employed.

Some individual hospitals have also published their experience with TH. For example, one hospital published its experience in developing and implementing a protocol to support induced hypothermia after cardiac arrest by a multidisciplinary team led by a neurointensivist.[60] Following this implementation, 25 patients were treated with TH. Of these patients, 74% survived, with 47% of these survivors discharged to home at the end of their hospitalization. Only 23% were transferred to a long-term care facility, with the remaining patients transferred to acute rehabilitation.

Similarly, Busch and colleagues[61] published their experience with rapid implementation of a simple TH protocol in comatose out-of-hospital SCA survivors. The protocol involved using prehospital cooling with ice packs in the groin and neck and ice water–soaked towels over the torso upon arrival in the ICU. The target temperature of 33 ± 1 °C was obtained in 24 of 27 patients (89%) with this simple cooling method. The hospital survival rate before and after the implementation of this protocol was compared. There was a higher survival rate in the patients who were treated with TH (59% versus 32%). A summary of selected TH clinical investigations and the randomized controlled trials supporting hypothermia is presented in **Table 1**.

Both of these experiences suggest that the implementation of a protocol may increase the appropriate use of TH following cardiac arrest. To improve post cardiac arrest care, several institutions have made their protocols available on the Internet (www.med.upenn.edu/resuscitation/hypothermia/).

TRAINING

Once a hospital develops a protocol for induced hypothermia, it must train its staff to ensure implementation. Unfortunately, there is no standardized course or method to train staff in the adoption and application of TH. The surveys discussed previously not only highlighted the need for standardized protocols but also pointed to the need for further education, because many physicians cited the lack of supporting evidence as one of the reasons for not using TH. Hospital training must include education to increase knowledge of the available trials and improved outcomes following cardiac arrests to ensure support of their protocols. Once knowledge is increased, mechanisms to practice the protocol and skills necessary to implement cooling must be in place.

Given a trend toward reduction in exposure of physicians-in-training to critically ill patients in the United States, simulation has been used more commonly to provide necessary instruction. In the medical domain, simulation methodology has historically focused on resuscitation, and many different tools are now being employed and developed, ranging from online simulation to integrated clinical simulators that use high-fidelity, whole-body manikins.[62] Simulation training may be used not only to identify the feasibility of proposed protocols but also to train health care staff in the implementation of such protocols and the technical skills necessary to cool a patient depending on the method used.

THERAPEUTIC HYPOTHERMIA FOR NEUROLOGIC INJURY AND OTHER APPLICATIONS

This review has focused on the use of hypothermia after resuscitation from cardiac arrest because the strongest data exist for this important application. An extensive literature has demonstrated that fever/hyperthermia is both common and deleterious in acute brain injury and stroke.[63,64] Furthermore, such fevers are generated from complex brain stem responses to neurologic insult and are hard to control with simple pharmacologic means such as acetaminophen. As such, the use of TH protocols and equipment to, at the very least, aggressively maintain normothermia is an evolving opportunity for treating the neurocritical patient. Several randomized controlled trials of TH in the setting of stroke are underway[65] and may offer hope to clinicians in the emergency department and neurocritical care unit. In areas where fever control is difficult, the beneficial effects of TH may have a role. These conditions typically include neurogenic fevers associated with acute neurologic injuries, such as stroke, and after subarachnoid hemorrhage or acute brain injuries.[63,66]

SUMMARY

After the accumulation of a large body of animal investigations of TH, two randomized controlled trials showed a benefit of induced hypothermia following out-of-hospital VF arrests in terms of survival and neurologic recovery.[19,20] This success led to recommendations by the ILCOR and AHA to induce mild-to-moderate hypothermia (32°C to 34°C) for 12 to 24 hours in any unconscious adult patient with ROSC after an out-of-hospital cardiac arrest and an initial rhythm of VF.[48] These recommendations state that such cooling may also be beneficial for other rhythms or in-hospital cardiac arrest. Additional work is ongoing to establish the potential neuroprotective benefit of TH for other disease processes such as stroke and neurotrauma. Several methods exist for cooling patients, and protocols for TH implementation are becoming more widely available. Through further dissemination of this important therapeutic option, patients sustaining ischemia-reperfusion injury and subsequent neurologic compromise may have a greater chance of leaving the hospital with improved function.

REFERENCES

1. Polderman KH. Application of therapeutic hypothermia in the ICU: opportunities and pitfalls of a promising treatment modality. Part 1. Indications and evidence. Intensive Care Med 2004;30(4):556–75.
2. Fay T. Observations on generalized refrigeration in cases of severe cerebral trauma. Assoc Res Nerv Ment Dis 1943;24:611–9.
3. Bigelow WC. Methods for inducing hypothermia and rewarming. Ann N Y Acad Sci 1959;80:522–32.
4. Bigelow WG, Callaghan JC, Hopps JA. General hypothermia for experimental intracardiac surgery: the use of electrophrenic respirations, an artificial pacemaker for cardiac standstill and radio-frequency rewarming in general hypothermia. Ann Surg 1950;132(3):531–9.
5. Botterell EH, Lougheed WM, Morley TP, et al. Hypothermia in the surgical treatment of ruptured intracranial aneurysms. J Neurosurg 1958;15(1):4–18.
6. Botterell EH, Lougheed WM, Scott JW, et al. Hypothermia and interruption of carotid, or carotid and vertebral circulation, in the surgical management of intracranial aneurysms. J Neurosurg 1956;13(1):1–42.

7. Curfman GD. Hypothermia to protect the brain. N Engl J Med 2002;346(8):546.
8. Marion DW, Leonov Y, Ginsberg M, et al. Resuscitative hypothermia. Crit Care Med 1996;24(2 Suppl):S81–9.
9. Eisenburger P, Sterz F, Holzer M, et al. Therapeutic hypothermia after cardiac arrest. Curr Opin Crit Care 2001;7(3):184–8.
10. Adams F. The genuine works of Hippocrates. New York: William Wood; 1886.
11. O'Sullivan ST, O'Shaughnessy M, O'Connor TP. Baron Larrey and cold injury during the campaigns of Napoleon. Ann Plast Surg 1995;34(4):446–9.
12. Safar P, Tisherman SA, Behringer W, et al. Suspended animation for delayed resuscitation from prolonged cardiac arrest that is unresuscitable by standard cardiopulmonary-cerebral resuscitation. Crit Care Med 2000;28(11 Suppl): N214–8.
13. Blair E, Henning G, Hornick R, et al. Hypothermia in bacteremic shock. Arch Surg 1964;89:619–29.
14. Safar P. Cerebral resuscitation after cardiac arrest: research initiatives and future directions. Ann Emerg Med 1993;22(2 Pt 2):324–49.
15. Benson DW, Williams GR Jr, Spencer FC, et al. The use of hypothermia after cardiac arrest. Anesth Analg 1959;38:423–8.
16. Ravitch MM, Lane R, Safar P, et al. Lightning stroke: report of a case with recovery after cardiac massage and prolonged artificial respiration. N Engl J Med 1961;264:36–8.
17. Gisvold SE, Safar P, Rao G, et al. Multifaceted therapy after global brain ischemia in monkeys. Stroke 1984;15(5):803–12.
18. Leonov Y, Sterz F, Safar P, et al. Moderate hypothermia after cardiac arrest of 17 minutes in dogs: effect on cerebral and cardiac outcome. Stroke 1990;21(11): 1600–6.
19. Bernard SA, Gray TW, Buist MD, et al. Treatment of comatose survivors of out-of-hospital cardiac arrest with induced hypothermia. N Engl J Med 2002;346(8): 557–63.
20. HACA study group. Mild therapeutic hypothermia to improve the neurologic outcome after cardiac arrest. N Engl J Med 2002;346(8):549–56.
21. Hachimi-Idrissi S, Corne L, Ebinger G, et al. Mild hypothermia induced by a helmet device: a clinical feasibility study. Resuscitation 2001;51(3):275–81.
22. Bernard S. Induced hypothermia in intensive care medicine. Anaesth Intensive Care 1996;24(3):382–8.
23. Colbourne F, Sutherland G, Corbett D. Postischemic hypothermia: a critical appraisal with implications for clinical treatment. Mol Neurobiol 1997;14(3): 171–201.
24. Coimbra C, Wieloch T. Moderate hypothermia mitigates neuronal damage in the rat brain when initiated several hours following transient cerebral ischemia. Acta Neuropathol 1994;87(4):325–31.
25. Colbourne F, Corbett D. Delayed and prolonged post-ischemic hypothermia is neuroprotective in the gerbil. Brain Res 1994;654(2):265–72.
26. Colbourne F, Li H, Buchan AM. Indefatigable CA1 sector neuroprotection with mild hypothermia induced 6 hours after severe forebrain ischemia in rats. J Cereb Blood Flow Metab 1999;19(7):742–9.
27. Hicks SD, DeFranco DB, Callaway CW. Hypothermia during reperfusion after asphyxial cardiac arrest improves functional recovery and selectively alters stress-induced protein expression. J Cereb Blood Flow Metab 2000;20(3): 520–30.

28. Hicks SD, Parmele KT, DeFranco DB, et al. Hypothermia differentially increases extracellular signal-regulated kinase and stress-activated protein kinase/c-Jun terminal kinase activation in the hippocampus during reperfusion after asphyxial cardiac arrest. Neuroscience 2000;98(4):677–85.

29. Zar HA, Lancaster JR Jr. Mild hypothermia protects against postischemic hepatic endothelial injury and decreases the formation of reactive oxygen species. Redox Rep 2000;5(5):303–10.

30. Markarian GZ, Lee JH, Stein DJ, et al. Mild hypothermia: therapeutic window after experimental cerebral ischemia. Neurosurgery 1996;38(3):542–50.

31. Behringer W, Prueckner S, Kentner R, et al. Rapid hypothermic aortic flush can achieve survival without brain damage after 30 minutes cardiac arrest in dogs. Anesthesiology 2000;93(6):1491–9.

32. Laptook AR, Corbett RJ, Sterett R, et al. Modest hypothermia provides partial neuroprotection when used for immediate resuscitation after brain ischemia. Pediatr Res 1997;42(1):17–23.

33. Woods RJ, Prueckner S, Safar P, et al. Hypothermic aortic arch flush for preservation during exsanguination cardiac arrest of 15 minutes in dogs. J Trauma 1999;47(6):1028–36.

34. Safar P, Xiao F, Radovsky A, et al. Improved cerebral resuscitation from cardiac arrest in dogs with mild hypothermia plus blood flow promotion. Stroke 1996; 27(1):105–13.

35. Weinrauch V, Safar P, Tisherman S, et al. Beneficial effect of mild hypothermia and detrimental effect of deep hypothermia after cardiac arrest in dogs. Stroke 1992;23(10):1454–62.

36. Nolan JP, Morley PT, Vanden Hoek TL, et al. Therapeutic hypothermia after cardiac arrest: an advisory statement by the advanced life support task force of the International Liaison Committee on Resuscitation. Circulation 2003;108(1): 118–21.

37. Jia X, Koenig MA, Shin HC, et al. Improving neurological outcomes post-cardiac arrest in a rat model: immediate hypothermia and quantitative EEG monitoring. Resuscitation 2008;76(3):431–42.

38. Oddo M, Schaller MD, Feihl F, et al. From evidence to clinical practice: effective implementation of therapeutic hypothermia to improve patient outcome after cardiac arrest. Crit Care Med 2006;34(7):1865–73.

39. Lawrence EJ, Dentcheva E, Curtis KM, et al. Neuroprotection with delayed initiation of prolonged hypothermia after in vitro transient global brain ischemia. Resuscitation 2005;64(3):383–8.

40. Wolfrum S, Radke PW, Pischon T, et al. Mild therapeutic hypothermia after cardiac arrest: a nationwide survey on the implementation of the ILCOR guidelines in German intensive care units. Resuscitation 2007;72(2):207–13.

41. Felberg RA, Krieger DW, Chuang R, et al. Hypothermia after cardiac arrest: feasibility and safety of an external cooling protocol. Circulation 2001;104(15): 1799–804.

42. Bernard S, Buist M, Monteiro O, et al. Induced hypothermia using large volume, ice-cold intravenous fluid in comatose survivors of out-of-hospital cardiac arrest: a preliminary report. Resuscitation 2003;56(1):9–13.

43. Merchant RM, Abella BS, Peberdy MA, et al. Therapeutic hypothermia after cardiac arrest: unintentional overcooling is common using ice packs and conventional cooling blankets. Crit Care Med 2006;34(12 Suppl): S490–4.

44. Xiao F, Safar P, Alexander H. Peritoneal cooling for mild cerebral hypothermia after cardiac arrest in dogs. Resuscitation 1995;30(1):51–9.

45. Inderbitzen B, Yon S, Lasheras J, et al. Safety and performance of a novel intravascular catheter for induction and reversal of hypothermia in a porcine model. Neurosurgery 2002;50(2):364–70.

46. Harris SB, Darwin MG, Russell SR, et al. Rapid (0.5°C/min) minimally invasive induction of hypothermia using cold perfluorochemical lung lavage in dogs. Resuscitation 2001;50(2):189–204.

47. Hong SB, Koh Y, Shim TS, et al. Physiologic characteristics of cold perfluorocarbon-induced hypothermia during partial liquid ventilation in normal rabbits. Anesth Analg 2002;94(1):157–62, table of contents.

48. Haugk M, Sterz F, Grassberger M, et al. Feasibility and efficacy of a new noninvasive surface cooling device in post-resuscitation intensive care medicine. Resuscitation 2007;75(1):76–81.

49. Al-Senani FM, Graffagnino C, Grotta JC, et al. A prospective, multicenter pilot study to evaluate the feasibility and safety of using the CoolGard System and Icy catheter following cardiac arrest. Resuscitation 2004;62(2):143–50.

50. Feuchtl A, Gockel B, Lawrenz T, et al. Endovascular cooling improves neurological short-term outcome after prehospital cardiac arrest. Intensivmedizin and Notfallmedizin [German] 2007;44:37–42.

51. Arpino PA, Greer DM. Practical pharmacologic aspects of therapeutic hypothermia after cardiac arrest. Pharmacotherapy 2008;28(1):102–11.

52. Polderman KH. Application of therapeutic hypothermia in the intensive care unit: opportunities and pitfalls of a promising treatment modality. Part 2. Practical aspects and side effects. Intensive Care Med 2004;30(5):757–69.

53. Aranda M, Hanson CW 3rd. Anesthetics, sedatives, and paralytics: understanding their use in the intensive care unit. Surg Clin North Am 2000;80(3):933–47.

54. 2005 American Heart Association guidelines for cardiopulmonary resuscitation and emergency cardiovascular care. Circulation 2005;112(24 Suppl):1–211.

55. Abella BS, Rhee JW, Huang KN, et al. Induced hypothermia is underused after resuscitation from cardiac arrest: a current practice survey. Resuscitation 2005; 64(2):181–6.

56. Merchant RM, Soar J, Skrifvars MB, et al. Therapeutic hypothermia utilization among physicians after resuscitation from cardiac arrest. Crit Care Med 2006; 34(7):1935–40.

57. Haque IU, Latour MC, Zaritsky AL. Pediatric critical care community survey of knowledge and attitudes toward therapeutic hypothermia in comatose children after cardiac arrest. Pediatr Crit Care Med 2006;7(1):7–14.

58. Majersik J, Silbergleit R, Meurer W, et al. Public health impact of full implementation of therapeutic hypothermia after cardiac arrest. Resuscitation 2008;77(2): 189–94.

59. Arrich J, ERC HACA study group. Clinical application of mild therapeutic hypothermia after cardiac arrest. Crit Care Med 2007;35(4):1041–7.

60. Cushman L, Warren ML, Livesay S. Bringing research to the bedside: the role of induced hypothermia in cardiac arrest. Crit Care Nurs Q 2007;30(2):143–53.

61. Busch M, Soreide E, Lossius HM, et al. Rapid implementation of therapeutic hypothermia in comatose out-of-hospital cardiac arrest survivors. Acta Anaesthesiol Scand 2006;50(10):1277–83.

62. Perkins GD. Simulation in resuscitation training. Resuscitation 2007;73(2): 202–11.

63. Fernandez A, Schmidt JM, Claassen J, et al. Fever after subarachnoid hemorrhage: risk factors and impact on outcome. Neurology 2007;68(13):1013–9.
64. Wong AA, Davis JP, Schluter PJ, et al. The time course and determinants of temperature within the first 48 h after ischaemic stroke. Cerebrovasc Dis 2007;24(1): 104–10.
65. Sacco RL, Chong JY, Prabhakaran S, et al. Experimental treatments for acute ischaemic stroke. Lancet 2007;369(9558):331–41.
66. Hoesch RE, Geocadin RG. Therapeutic hypothermia for global and focal ischemic brain injury: a cool way to improve neurologic outcomes. Neurologist 2007; 13(6):331–42.

Glycemic Control and the Injured Brain

Nina T. Gentile, MD[a],*, Karen Siren, MD[b]

KEYWORDS

- Hyperglycemia • Diabetes mellitus • Neurological illness

The interaction between glycemic control and critical neurologic illness and injury is complex. Hyperglycemia can be either the cause or the result of severe brain injury. Hyperglycemia in acute neurologic injury is associated with worse neurologic outcomes. Demographic patterns, including an aging population and shifts in racial and ethnic representation, contribute to the increasing prevalence of hyperglycemia and diabetes among victims of the most common neurologic emergencies. This article reviews the epidemiology of the problem, relevant pathophysiology, the use of tight glycemic control therapy in other populations, and the potential for tight glycemic control as a way to improve outcomes after acute neurologic illness and injury.

BURDEN OF ACUTE NEUROLOGIC DISEASE

Neurologic emergencies, including traumatic brain injury (TBI), seizure, and stroke (ischemic, intracranial hemorrhage, or subarachnoid hemorrhage), are among the most common and most lethal illnesses or injuries. Neurologic emergencies are among the most common causes for visits to emergency departments in the United States. Outcomes from these events vary from mild confusion to recurrent or prolonged disability and death. At times even mild or subtle symptoms such as headache or mental status changes can herald serious intracranial disease such as meningitis or venous sinus thrombosis.

Traumatic Brain Injury

Each year, an estimated 1.4 million persons sustain TBI,[1–3] most commonly from unintentional falls, motor vehicle accidents, and physical assault. The tremendously high rates of TBI from motor vehicle accidents among 15- to 19-year-olds is well known.[4] The Centers for Disease Control, however, recently reported a dramatic rise in the

---

[a] Department of Emergency Medicine, 1007 Jones Hall, 3401 North Broad Street, Temple University School of Medicine, Philadelphia, PA 19140, USA
[b] Emergency Medicine Residency Program, Temple University Hospital, Philadelphia, PA, USA
* Corresponding author.
E-mail address: ngentile@temple.edu (N.T. Gentie).

Emerg Med Clin N Am 27 (2009) 151–169
doi:10.1016/j.emc.2008.08.010
0733-8627/08/$ – see front matter © 2009 Elsevier Inc. All rights reserved.

emed.theclinics.com

TBI-related hospitalization rate (from 165 per 100,000 in 1997 to 264 per 100,000 population in 2002) in persons aged more than 75 years; these patients suffer TBI not from motor vehicle accidents but from unintentional falls.[5] The increasing age of the United States population is changing emergency department patient demographics with resultant increases in the incidence and severity of neurologic disease and injury. The rise in the incidence of spinal cord injury and posttraumatic seizure in older patients parallels the increases in the rate of TBI.[6]

Seizure Disorder

Although epilepsy usually is idiopathic, the risk of developing seizure after TBI is greater than 3% after a mild closed head injury and is 15% after severe TBI, rates much higher than the 0.5% to 1% risk in the general population.[6] After penetrating head injury, the incidence of seizure is as high as 53%.[7]

The risk of developing seizure is highest in conditions that lead to injury or dysfunction of the cerebral cortex. The risk of developing seizures is high in patients who have experienced hemorrhagic stroke, penetrating head injury, or are withdrawing from alcohol or drug abuse. These conditions occur more often in poorer, often urban-dwelling, minority populations and may explain the high rates of seizure disorder in these communities.[8]

Stroke

Stroke is the third leading cause of death and is the primary cause of acquired physical disability in the United States.[9] Up to a third of patients remain functionally dependent 1 year after the stroke, and the need for long-term medical care or institutionalization[10] results in considerable health care costs. In the United States, stroke costs more than $56.8 billion annually, 62% of which is accounted for by hospital and home care costs.[11]

NEUROEMERGENCIES IN MINORITY POPULATIONS

Special issues need to be considered with regard to the diagnosis and treatment of neuroemergencies in minority populations.

Traumatic: Role of Brain Injury Drugs, Alcohol, and Violence

The types and causes of TBI in urban, primarily African American and Hispanic, communities are different from those in suburban or rural communities.[12] Motor vehicle accidents account for the majority of TBIs outside the city; urban patients suffer head injuries from assaults that often involve the use of firearms and from falls. Firearms are the single largest cause of death from TBI in the United States, and the devastating TBIs caused by bullet wounds result in a 91% death rate for firearm-related TBIs overall.[13] African Americans have a much greater risk of dying from firearm-related TBI than do people of other races. No matter the cause of TBI, African American and Hispanic patients are less likely to receive physical or vocational rehabilitation or psychologic counseling[14] and are less functionally independent 1 year after injury.[15] **Fig. 1** shows TBI-related death rates by cause and race in the United States in 1994.

High Prevalence of Stroke and Cerebrovascular Disease

Each year, 700,000 people suffer a new or recurrent stroke, and stroke accounts for 1 of every 15 deaths. Stroke is one of the leading causes of disability, and the public health burden of stroke falls more heavily on select groups such as African Americans between the ages of 35 and 65 years.[11] The prevalence of risk factors for

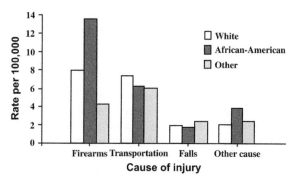

Fig. 1. Traumatic brain injury–related death rates by cause and race in the United States, 1994.

cerebrovascular disease is highest among African Americans (**Table 1**).[16] Diabetes and obesity, known to be independent predictors of mortality after stroke,[17] are particularly prevalent among African American and Hispanic women.

Racial Differences in Stroke Mortality Rates

Several population-based studies, such as the Northern Manhattan Stroke Study,[18] the Rochester, MN,[19] and the Greater Cincinnati/Northern Kentucky Stroke Study,[20] have demonstrated a significant racial disparity in all-type stroke incidence rates and risk factors among different racial and ethnic groups. Also, there are differences in treatment[21] and in response to treatment[22] among racial and ethnic groups. For example, among patients seeking treatment for an ischemic stroke, intravenous tissue plasminogen activator is used less frequently in African American patients presenting within 3 hours of symptom onset.[21] Moreover, despite insulin and oral blood

Table 1
Prevalence of risk factors by race/ethnicity and sex for cardiovascular disease in the United States

Risk Factors and Conditions	Non-Hispanic Whites Males	Non-Hispanic Whites Females	African Americans Males	African Americans Females	Mexican Americans Males	Mexican Americans Females
High blood pressure[a]	25.2	20.5	36.7	36.6	24.2	22.4
High LDL-cholesterol[b]	49.6	43.7	46.3	41.6	43.6	41.6
Smoking[c]	25.8	21.6	26.1	20.8	24.1	12.3
Physical Inactivity[d]	32.5	36.2	44.1	55.2	48.9	57.4
Obesity[e]	27.3	30.1	28.1	49.7	28.9	39.7
Diabetes[f]	5.4	4.7	7.6	9.5	8.1	11.4

[a] Systolic blood pressure ≥ 140 mm Hg; diastolic blood pressure ≥ 90 mm Hg, or patient taking anti-hypertensive medication; age adjusted for people age 20 years and older.
[b] Low-density lipoprotein cholesterol ≥ 130 mg/dL; age adjusted for people age 20 years and older.
[c] In people age 18 years and older.
[d] No leisure-time activity in people age 18 years and older.
[e] Body mass index ≥ 30 kg/m² in people age 20 and older.
[f] Physician-diagnosed diabetes; age adjusted for people age 20 and older.
Data from American Heart Association. Heart and stroke statistics—2003 update. Dallas (TX): American Heart Association; 2002; with permission.

glucose–lowering medications, African American and Hispanic patients suffering acute ischemic stroke who have type 2 diabetes mellitus are more likely than whites to have persistent, uncontrolled hyperglycemia.[22]

THE DIABETES EPIDEMIC

The crude prevalence of total diabetes in the period from 1999 to 2002 was 9.3% (19.3 million, 2002 United States population), of which 6.5% was diagnosed and 2.8% was undiagnosed. An additional 26.0% of the population had impaired fasting glucose levels, so 35.3% of the population (73.3 million people) had either diabetes or impaired fasting glucose levels. The prevalence of diabetes rose with age, reaching 21.6% for those age 65 years and older. The prevalence of diagnosed diabetes was twice as high in Hispanics and non-Hispanic blacks (both $P<.00001$) than in non-Hispanic whites.[23]

Diabetes in Minority Populations

Although diabetes has a major adverse impact on life years and quality-adjusted life years in all United States subpopulations, the impact is even greater among minority individuals, including African Americans and Hispanics. Ethnic minorities in the United States are disproportionately affected by diabetes-related complications including diabetic retinopathy, lower extremity amputation, and end-stage renal disease.[24–27] Among patients who have had ischemic stroke, Hispanics have the highest rate of diabetes, and this increased rate of diabetes may the reason poststroke mortality is four times higher in Hispanic patients than in non-Hispanic patients.[16]

HYPERGLYCEMIA IN ACUTE ILLNESS AND INJURY

Disturbances in glucose and cortisol homeostasis during critical illness are well known.[28,29] Whether pre-existing or illness/injury-related, electrolyte or metabolic derangements and endocrinopathies, if left unattended, may lead to significant morbidity and mortality. Many of these alterations are in fact homeostatic corrections that result from finely tuned, complex, and often multisystemic evolutionary adaptations for coping with the catastrophic events during critical illness. There is evidence for the presence of an orchestrated endocrine, immune, and nervous system response to inflammation. In addition to the release of cortisol and thyroid hormone, levels of endocrine humoral substances such as arachidonic acids, nitric oxide, endothelin, leptin, and adenosine rise in acute illness and injury. Furthermore the "hormokines" procalcitonin and adrenomedullin are released during inflammation with levels that increase several 10,000-fold during sepsis.[28] These cytokine-like compounds serve as immune markers correlating with injury severity and outcome. Whereas most acute-phase proteins, such as C-reactive protein and serum amyloid A, are highly sensitive to inflammatory activity and can be important markers of severity and outcome, some (eg, natriuretic peptides) are more system specific.[29] Although measuring neurocrine and hormokine biomarkers can improve clinical acumen and help guide treatment, these compounds also act as inflammatory mediators. Like all mediators, their role during illness or injury is basically beneficial, but at higher levels they can become harmful, and their role in critical illness is less clear.[30]

Hyperglycemia in Stroke

Hyperglycemia is common in patients who have had an acute stroke. The rate of concomitant hyperglycemia in acute stroke is estimated to be between 25% and 50% but was reported to be as high as 68% in one series.[31] Hyperglycemic patients who have suffered an acute stroke have worse postischemic brain injury and cerebral edema and poorer outcomes than patients who have normal blood glucose levels after stroke.[32–35] Even slightly elevated blood glucose levels of 125 to 130 mg/dL have been associated with a longer hospital length of stay, higher mortality rate,[36] and increased infarct volume on MRI.[37] Acute hyperglycemia has been associated with hemorrhagic transformation of an infarct in animal experiments[38–40] and in two clinical reports.[41,42]

The effects of hyperglycemia in acute stroke depend on the presence of diabetes mellitus, on whether the tissue is reperfused, and on the stroke subtype. Hyperglycemia occurs in patients who have diabetes mellitus; and it can occur in patients who do not have diabetes as a result of an early hormonal response to cerebral ischemia. Some studies have suggested that hyperglycemia in acute stroke is more detrimental in patients who have diabetes mellitus.[37] Others have suggested that hyperglycemia after an acute stroke in patients who do not have diabetes mellitus is stress induced and portends a poorer outcome than in diabetic patients.[31] In a systematic review of observational studies examining the prognostic significance of hyperglycemia in acute stroke, the relative risk of death after ischemic stroke in patients who had admission blood glucose levels higher than 110 to 126 mg/dL was 3.28 overall. In addition to the greater risk of poor functional recovery, the unadjusted relative risk of in-hospital or 30-day mortality was 3.07 (95% confidence interval [CI], 2.50–3.79) in nondiabetic patients and 1.30 (95% CI, 0.49–3.43) in patients who had diabetes.[31] Reactive or stress hyperglycemia has been attributed to the activation of the hypothalamic-pituitary-adrenal axis and the sympathoadrenal systems,[43–45] leading to increased circulating cortisol and catecholamines. Reactive hyperglycemia is related to stroke severity and is unlikely in patients who have had a lacunar stroke.[46] Larger strokes may cause both an acutely elevated blood glucose level and a worse outcome. Although few studies have controlled for stroke size and severity, an analysis that controlled for stroke severity suggests that although acute hyperglycemia may be a response to stroke, it augments brain injury in both lacunar and nonlacunar stroke.[31]

Patients who have type 2 diabetes mellitus are likely to have microvascular and atherosclerotic disease that leads to lacunar, atherothrombotic, and (albeit to a lesser extent) cardioembolic stroke. Mortality rates vary by stroke subtype; 1-year mortality rates range from 14% to 45%, and 2-year mortality rates rise to 28% after lacunar stroke and to more than 60% after cardioembolic stroke.[47] Recurrent stroke rates, approximately 15% to 20% during the year following stroke, are highest in patients who have lacunar and atherosclerotic stroke.[48–50] Diabetes is one of the best predictors of stroke recurrence,[48] increasing the risk of recurrent stroke by at least 35%,[48] and persistent hyperglycemia doubles the rate of recurrent stroke.[51]

The degree to which blood glucose is maintained in a relatively normal range affects mortality after acute stroke. Patients who have persistent euglycemia have much lower mortality rates than persistently hyperglycemic patients, and normalization of blood glucose early after stroke is a strong independent determinant of survival (odds ratio [OR], 5.95; 95% CI, 1.24–28.6; $P = .026$), even after adjustment for age, gender, concomitant hypertension and diabetes, and stroke severity (**Table 2**).[51]

Hyperglycemia in Subarachnoid Hemorrhage

Hyperglycemia may predispose to poor outcome after aneurysmal subarachnoid hemorrhage (SAH). Patients who have had SAH and who have even transient episodes of perioperative hyperglycemia are seven- to 10-fold more likely to have a poorer outcome (ie, be functionally dependent) than patients who have normal blood glucose levels, independent of admission Hunt and Hess grade, occurrence of cerebral vasospasm, or comorbidities.[52] Patients who had the highest serum glucose levels had the

Table 2
Mortality rates by glycemic control groups

	Glycemic Control Group		
Patient disposition	Persistent euglycemia (N=396)	Persistent hyperglycemia (N=246)	χ^2 or F-value
Mortality	5 (1.3%)	19 (7.7%)	18.9 ($P = .001$)

Data from Gentile NT, Seftcheck M, Matonti M, et al. Decreased mortality with normalizing blood glucose after acute stroke. Acad Emerg Med 2006;13:174–80.

lowest extracellular fluid glucose concentrations and the highest levels of anaerobic metabolites, lactate, lactate/pyruvate ratio, and lactate/glucose ratio, indicating cerebral metabolic distress.[53]

Hyperglycemia in Meningitis

Unlike patients who have had an acute stroke and SAH, clinical studies of patients who have hyperglycemia and bacterial meningitis have shown mixed results. Some studies show that the intensity and duration of hyperglycemia are associated with poorer outcomes in critically ill children who have meningococcemia.[54] In one study, children who had septic shock had a 2.6-fold rise in mortality when peak glucose levels exceeded 178 mg/dL.[55] Other studies have shown no association between initial serum glucose concentration and subsequent mortality with meningitis.

In fact, some suggest that patients who have bacterial meningitis might benefit from induced hyperglycemia to increase glucose delivery to meet the demands of an increased cerebral glycolytic rate.[56] The mechanism of a putative beneficial effect of induced hyperglycemia in meningitis is not clear at present. One thought is that the abnormally low concentration of glucose in the cerebrospinal fluid (CSF) observed in patients who have meningitis may result in a condition akin to systemic hypoglycemia. Systemic hypoglycemia is correlated with decreases in brain glucose levels, cerebral oxidative metabolism, and in the synthesis of high-energy phosphate compounds. ATP depletion during hypoglycemia leads to decreased re-uptake of energy-dependent excitotoxic amino acids (EAA). This decreased re-upake leads to toxic EAA accumulation with resultant neuronal death.[57] Hypoglycorrhachia (low CSF glucose) observed even in meningitic patients who have systemic normoglycemia may lead to neuronal death by similar mechanisms. If so, induced hyperglycemia could correct this relative insufficiency of brain glucose and might be beneficial by providing an increased glucose delivery to meet the brain's increased demand and might reduce excitotoxicity by increasing neuronal EAA re-uptake. In addition, elevated glucose concentration could provide additional substrate NADPH for maintenance of the pool of reduced glutathione, which functions as an oxygen free radical scavenger. Glutathione acts to repair oxidant injury in cell membranes by undergoing oxidation while reducing lipid peroxidation products that have been formed by oxygen free radicals. Reduced lipid peroxidation products observed in hyperglycemic patients who have meningitis support this assumption.[57]

PATHOPHYSIOLOGY OF HYPERGLYCEMIC INJURY IN CRITICAL ILLNESS

The acute phase of critical illness usually is characterized by hyperglycemia. Hyperglycemia during critical illness is induced by both increased glucose production and decreased glucose cellular uptake (**Fig. 2**). High levels of glucose are produced

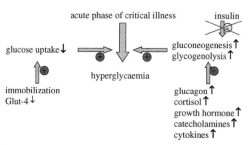

Fig. 2. Potential mechanisms for the induction of hyperglycemia in critical illness and injury.

through up-regulation of both gluconeogenesis and glycogenolysis. In addition, illness-related increases in cortisol, catecholamine, and cytokine levels induce hyperglycemia in acute injury. Cellular glucose uptake is severely diminished in critical injury and illness. Insulin regulates glucose uptake by altering the distribution of the facilitative glucose transporter Glut 4 in muscle, fat, and cardiac cells. In normal conditions, 80% of glucose clearance is by uptake into skeletal muscle through exercise. Largely because of immobility in the very ill, normal exercise-induced insulin-stimulated glucose uptake into skeletal muscle is almost completely absent. Therefore, glucose is not cleared despite very high levels of insulin, a condition akin to insulin resistance. Normal cells respond to moderate hyperglycemia by down-regulating glucose transporters to protect themselves from the deleterious effects of high glucose. Unlike Glut 4, however, the glucose transporters Glut 1, Glut 2, and Glut 3 are insulin independent. These transporters allow the entry of excess glucose into cells of the central and peripheral nervous system, hepatocytes, renal tubules, gastrointestinal mucosa, endothelial cells, and the immune system. In critical illness, hypoxia, or other conditions with elevated acute-phase reactants (such as cytokines, angiotensin II, or endothelin I), Glut 1 and Glut 3 receptor expression and activity are increased, resulting in intracellular glucose accumulation.

Mechanisms of Hyperglycemia-Induced Brain Injury

Hyperglycemia affects multiple microvascular and cellular pathways and contributes to pathologic changes after acute stroke. The most consistent findings linking hyperglycemia to brain damage in experimental stroke are acidosis[58,59] and excitatory amino acid production.[60,61] During an ischemic event, local increases in anaerobic glycolysis are associated with intracellular acidosis occurring shortly after the ischemic insult. Animals with acute hyperglycemia develop acidic mean cortical pH as well as high cerebral lactate concentrations, leading to neuronal and glial damage.[58,59] Excitatory amino acids, most notably glutamate, play a central role in neuronal death by the activation of postsynaptic glutamate receptors.[60,61] This activation leads to an excessive influx of calcium through ion channels, mitochondrial injury, and eventual cell death. Hyperglycemia exaggerates edema formation,[62] injury to the blood–brain barrier,[63] and hemorrhagic transformation of the infarct. In a model of middle cerebral artery occlusion, a fivefold increase in hemorrhagic infarct and a 25-fold increase in extensive hemorrhages were observed in hyperglycemic cats compared with the normoglycemic animals.[38]

Tissue factor–dependent coagulation and subsequent thrombosis play a major role in acute vascular events, especially in patients who have diabetes mellitus. Patients who have had an acute ischemic stroke may be in a hypercoagulable state, in part because of activation of the tissue factor pathway. Hyperglycemia contributes to this effect by activating blood coagulation mechanisms leading to increased thrombin generation, as evidenced by elevated Factor VIIa, a precursor for thrombin-antithrombin activation.[64]

Insulin and glycemic control protect against thrombogenesis by reducing tissue factor–induced elevations in Factor VIIa and by reducing fibrinogen and plasminogen activator inhibitor (PAI)-1 levels.[65] Intensive insulin treatment lowers C-reactive protein and serum amyloid A levels and induces a profibrinolytic effect by attenuating the rise in PAI-1 after thrombolysis for acute myocardial infarction.[65]

Mechanisms of the Beneficial Effect of Insulin in Acute Neurologic Injury

The effects of endogenous insulin therapy in acute neurologic pathology potentially are mediated by direct neuroprotective effects in the brain or by systemic metabolic effects. In addition to its systemic effects, insulin can enter the brain and act as a potent neuropeptide, which has been shown to reduce ischemic brain and spinal cord damage. Studies that have controlled for glucose levels have shown that insulin acts directly on the neurons and glia, independent of hypoglycemia, to reduce ischemic brain necrosis.[66] Possible direct central nervous system mechanisms of action include an effect on central insulin receptors mediating inhibitory neuromodulation,[67] an effect on central neurotransmitters, or a growth factor effect of insulin.[68]

Exogenous insulin also simply can enforce euglycemia systemically and attenuate the effects of hyperglycemic injury mechanisms. Evidence in favor of this simple mechanism includes data from Finney and colleagues[69] showing that in critically ill patients the mortality benefit correlates more closely with the adequacy of blood glucose control than with the dose of exogenous insulin administered.

Both direct and indirect mechanisms probably are contributory, and the role of each may vary with the type of neurologic injury. In animal models, insulin alters neurologic functional outcome and mortality after global injury (eg, after cardiac arrest) primarily by its central neuroprotective effects, but after focal brain injury, such as stroke, the benefit is obtained predominantly through the lowering of systemic blood glucose.[66–68,70,71]

TIGHT GLYCEMIC CONTROL IN GENERAL CRITICAL CARE AND NEUROEMERGENCIES

The benefits of controlling blood glucose levels with insulin in acutely ill patients have emerged in recent years. The use of insulin protocols improves the control of blood glucose levels and reduces morbidity and mortality in critically ill populations. Several randomized clinical trials have indicated benefit from short-term strict glucose control in hospitalized patients,[72–74] during general surgical and postoperative care,[75] and after acute myocardial infarction.[76] The positive results of clinical trials on insulin infusion therapy in other acute conditions have rekindled interest in the possible therapeutic efficacy of insulin in hyperglycemia associated with acute neurologic emergencies.

Coronary Artery Surgery

Hyperglycemic patients undergoing cardiac surgery suffer greater mortality, more deep wound infections, and overall higher rates of infection than patients who have normal blood glucose levels.[77] Postoperative hyperglycemia is an important predictor for infection and mortality in both diabetic and nondiabetic patients.[78]

The Portland protocol was one of the earliest experiences in using large-scale continuous insulin infusion to manage hyperglycemia aggressively in the hospital setting.[79] The protocol was implemented in gradual steps designed to maintain patient safety, prevent hypoglycemia, and ensure nursing comfort and compliance. The protocol was used first in 1992 with a target blood glucose range of 150 to 200 mg/dL in the ICUs only. In 1996, the protocol was expanded with initiation in the operating room and continuation on the telemetry floor until the third postoperative day. Target blood glucose levels gradually were lowered to 125 to 175 mg/dL in 1999 and then to 100 to 150 mg/dL in 2001. **Fig. 3** shows the average postoperative glucose levels of 3554 diabetic patients after coronary artery bypass graft surgery from 1986 to 2002.[80]

Glucose control using continuous insulin infusion is associated with a dramatically decreased incidence of wound infection and mortality in patients after cardiac surgery. The rate of deep wound infection dropped from 67% to 25% to 13% when blood glucose levels decreased from 250 to 300 mg/dL, to 200 to 250 mg/dL, and then to 100 to 150 mg/dL, respectively.[77,79] Treatment with insulin infusion led to a significantly lower mortality (2.5%) than seen with subcutaneous insulin (5.3%) and was shown to be independently protective against death (OR, 0.43).

Acute Myocardial Infarction

In 1995, the Diabetes and Insulin-Glucose Infusion in Acute Myocardial Infarction (DIGAMI) study was the first to assign diabetic patients who had acute myocardial infarction randomly to either intensive insulin therapy or standard treatment.[81] Intensive insulin therapy consisted of intravenous infusion of glucose-insulin-potassium (GIK) as soon as possible after the acute myocardial infarction and continued for 48 hours. Thereafter, patients in the intensive insulin therapy group were submitted to a stricter regimen of blood glucose control with subcutaneous insulin continued for 3 months after discharge. In the intensive treatment arm, mortality risk at 1 year was reduced by a relative 29%.[81] In addition, there was a significant decrease in reinfarction and new heart failure. It remained unclear, however, how much of the benefit resulted from an acute effect of GIK and how much was mediated by strict blood glucose control with insulin in the days and months after the acute myocardial infarction.

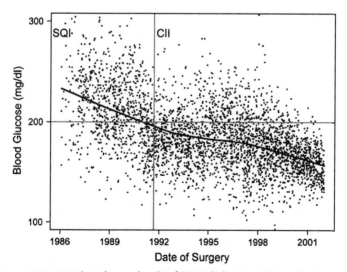

Fig. 3. Average postoperative glucose levels of 3554 diabetic patients after coronary artery bypass graft surgery from 1986 to 2002. (*Data from* Furnary AP, Zerr KJ, Grunkemeier GL, et al. Hyperglycemia: a predictor of mortality following CABG in diabetics. Circulation 1999;100:1–591.)

A follow-up to the DAGMI 1 trial studied the short-term and long-term effects of intensive insulin treatment in patients who had acute myocardial infarction and diabetes.[82] Subjects were assigned randomly to either continued management as determined by their physicians or to intravenous infusion of insulin and glucose for 48 hours followed by a four-injection regimen (subcutaneous insulin administered four times daily) for as long as 5 years. Most of the benefit was apparent in the first month of treatment and presumably resulted in part from the immediate intravenous infusion of insulin; however, the survival curves tended to separate further over time, suggesting an ongoing benefit from intensive treatment.

A later study, DIGAMI 2, unlike DAGAMI 1, did not find that an acutely introduced, long-term insulin treatment improves survival after myocardial infarction in patients who have type 2 diabetes when compared with conventional management at similar levels of glucose control or that insulin-based treatment lowers the number of nonfatal myocardial re-infarctions and strokes.[83] In contrast with DAGMI 1, however, the patients in the different treatment groups in DIGAMI 2 did not differ in blood glucose level or A1c. With the exception of differences found in 24-hour blood glucose levels and 3-day A1c levels, there were no differences in glucose or A1c levels between treatment groups. This lack of difference may explain the observed lack of effect in DIGAMI 2 as compared with DIGAMI 1.

Studies of glycemic control in patients who have had an acute myocardial infarction underscore the importance of avoiding hypoglycemia during intensive insulin therapy. There is a U-shaped relationship between blood glucose levels and adverse outcomes among patients who have ST-segment elevation acute myocardial infarction. Patients who have high Thrombosis in Myocardial Infarction (TIMI) risk scores (> 4) after acute myocardial infarction and blood glucose levels higher than 150 mg/dL or lower than 81 mg/dL are at greater risk for adverse events than patients who have TIMI risk scores between 0 and 4 or whose blood glucose levels are between 81 and 125 mg/dL.[84]

Surgical Critical Care

One of the earliest and most definitive randomized, controlled studies of strict glycemic control was performed in surgical ICU patients. A heterogeneous group of 1548 patients was enrolled and assigned randomly to receive conventional therapy or intravenous insulin by continuous infusion for blood glucose management.[72] Patients were enrolled if their blood glucose levels exceeded 110 mg/dL. The goal of intensive therapy was to keep the blood glucose level between 80 and 110 mg/dL. The target for conventional therapy was a blood glucose level between 180 and 200 mg/dL. In this study, meticulous glycemic control with insulin infusion led to a dramatic reduction in risk for ICU mortality (42%); sepsis (46%); need for dialysis (41%), blood transfusion (50%), and ventilatory support (39%).[72] Results of the trial demonstrated an impressive improvement in postsurgical survival with intensive glycemic control. Moreover, the mortality benefit in these critically ill patients seems to be related to the control of the blood glucose level rather than to the amount of exogenous insulin given.[69]

In critically injured trauma patients, hyperglycemia (moderate, worsening, and highly variable) is associated with significantly greater hospital and ICU length of stay, ventilator time, infection, and mortality after controlling for age, race, gender, injury severity score, mechanism of injury, obesity, and insulin-dependent diabetes.[85] Implementation of a tight glucose control protocol during the first week of admission in critically injured trauma patients has reduced significantly the incidence of infection, the number of days of mechanical ventilation, ICU length of stay, hospital length of stay, and mortality.[86]

Medical Critical Care

Even before definitive studies were performed to substantiate its use, intensive insulin therapy was widely advocated during critical illness with severe sepsis.[87] During the past 7 years, evidence has emerged suggesting that glycemic control in the medical ICU setting improves outcome when (1) patients are critically ill (ie, require an ICU stay $\geq$ 3 days) and (2) hypoglycemia is avoided. Using the same Leuven titration protocol described earlier,[72] van den Berghe, and colleagues[73] found less impressive differences between intensive insulin and conventional therapy in medical ICU patients than in surgical ICU patients. Among the 1200 patients assigned to conventional therapy or intensive blood glucose treatment in the medical ICU, intensive insulin therapy had no beneficial effect on overall survival rates.[73] In the subset of patients who had stayed in the ICU for 3 or more days, however, in-hospital mortality was significantly reduced (from 52.5% to 43.0%) with intensive insulin therapy, as was morbidity (multisystem dysfunction, need for mechanical ventilation). Also, in this study, intensive therapy was associated with a five- to sixfold increase in hypoglycemic events (mean glucose level, 31 mg/dL), and such events probably contributed to the negative findings related to intensive insulin in the medical ICU setting.

Neurologic Critical Care

Relatively few prospective studies of glycemic control have included patients who had acute neurologic injury or illness. Post hoc analysis of 63 patients who had isolated brain injury from the larger Leuven cohort of surgical ICU patients examined the effect of insulin therapy on intracranial pressure, diabetes insipidus, seizures, and long-term rehabilitation at 6 and 12 months' follow-up. Both neurologic and non-neurologic morbidity were reduced in the group treated with insulin infusion.[87]

Traumatic brain injury

Hyperglycemia also has been studied as an important outcome indicator in TBI. Jeremitsky and colleagues[88] found that hyperglycemia was associated with increased mortality and longer hospital stays. In another study of patients who had suffered TBI, high glucose levels on admission were associated with worsened neurologic outcomes.[89] One small study targeting patients who had acute TBI found that intensive insulin therapy resulted in a net reduction in microdialysis glucose levels.[90] Despite a reduction in microdialysis glucose, intensive insulin therapy was associated with increased global oxygen extraction fraction and increased incidence of microdialysis markers of cellular distress including elevations in glutamate and lactate/pyruvate ratio. Functionally, patients in this study had similar mortality rates and 6-month clinical outcomes regardless of blood glucose control.[90]

Acute ischemic stroke

Hyperglycemia is known to be detrimental to outcome after stroke, and lowering blood glucose to near normal levels has been associated with reduced morbidity and mortality. Nonetheless, the effects of insulin after acute ischemic stroke still are not clear. Retrospectively reviewed data of 960 patients who had stroke showed that hyperglycemia on hospital admission was associated with a higher mortality rate than euglycemia (OR, 3.15).[51] Glycemic control (normalization of blood glucose) was associated with a nearly sevenfold reduction in absolute mortality rate compared with patients who had persistent hyperglycemia over 48 hours of hospitalization. Glycemic control was a strong independent determinant of survival (OR, 8.52) after acute stroke, even after adjustment for age, gender, concomitant hypertension and diabetes, and stroke severity.[51] These findings are limited, however, by the retrospective design of the study.

There have been multiple reports that insulin can reduce neuronal damage, improve functional outcome, reduce the area of infarction, and reduce mortality in experimental models of acute ischemic brain injury,[91–93] but only two prospective clinical studies have assessed the efficacy of insulin infusion therapy in acute stroke.[94,95] In the first study, a GIK infusion was used to treat patients who had mild or moderate hypoglycemia (average serum glucose level, 160 mg/dL). The investigators found no difference between patients treated with GIK and those treated with standard therapy.[94] One hypothesis for this lack of effect is that, because the effect of insulin in stroke is predominantly via peripheral hypoglycemia rather than by its central neuroprotective effects,[66–68,70,71] the glucose in the GIK solution may have canceled the potential beneficial effects of the insulin.

The UK Glucose Insulin Stroke Trial[95] was a randomized study comparing GIK infusion with control (normal saline) in patients who had suffered an acute stroke and had blood glucose levels between 110 and 300 mg/dL. The target blood glucose level was between 75 and 125 mg/dL, and the primary end point was mortality at day 90. In this study, mortality rates were similar in the two groups: 30% in the treated and 27.3% in the control group. Several factors may have played a role in the neutral results.[96] First, treatment with GKI was associated with significant decreases in blood pressure, with a mean fall in systolic blood pressure of 9.03 mm Hg. Second, despite a glucose enrollment range of 110 to 300 mg/dL, most of the recruited patients had mild hyperglycemia with median blood glucose levels of 140.4 mg/dL (range, 122.4–165.6 mg/dL) in the GKI group and 136.8 mg/dL (range, 120.6–158.4 mg/dL) in the placebo group. In this study, as in the study by Scott and colleagues,[94] average posttreatment blood glucose levels in the two groups were similar. In this study, the glucose concentration fell spontaneously with intravenous saline alone.

Several studies have been reported or are ongoing to determine the feasibility and safety of insulin infusion titrated to achieve a target glucose concentration after acute ischemic stroke.[97–101] In one study, insulin infusion effectively brought down the blood glucose level from a mean of 270 mg/dL to 131 $\pm$ 19.8 mg/dL.[98] However, at least one episode of hypoglycemia occurred in 11 of 24 patients (46%), and 5 of these patients (21%) had symptomatic hypoglycemia.[101] A more recent study by the same group[102] showed that aggressive insulin therapy can achieve a target blood glucose level (< 130 mg/dL) within about 4 hours after initiation with an overall rate of mostly asymptomatic hypoglycemia (blood glucose level < 60 mg/dL) of 35%.[103]

THE NUTS AND BOLTS OF INSULIN PROTOCOLS

At the core of optimal blood glucose management after illness or injury are early insulin administration and frequent monitoring and regulation of blood glucose levels. The best strategy for controlling blood glucose is the use of an insulin infusion protocol. Such approaches, however, are labor intensive, expensive, and often inconsistently applied. In-hospital resources often are limited, especially outside the ICU setting, and intensive blood glucose control is given a low priority in the care of patients who have acute neurologic emergencies.

Comparison of Insulin Protocols

There is large variability among insulin protocols. Areas of variation include differences in initiation and titration of insulin, use of bolus dosing, requirements for calculation in adjustment of the insulin infusion, and method of insulin protocol adjustments. The amount of time needed to reach the target range varies greatly among protocols as does the range of insulin dose recommended (range, 27–115 units; mean ± SD, 66.7 ± 27.9).[101] Based on experience using insulin protocols and the outcomes of multiple retrospective and prospective studies, the American Diabetes Association and the American College of Endocrinology have made recommendations regarding the degree of blood glucose management in both the ICU and the general ward settings (**Table 3**).[103]

Hypoglycemia in Blood Glucose Management

Recent studies emphasize the need to avoid hypoglycemia during blood glucose management in critical illness.[102] A recent multicenter trial comparing intensive insulin therapy with conventional treatment to maintain euglycemia in patients who had severe sepsis was stopped early for safety reasons. Among 537 patients who could be evaluated, there was no significant difference between the two groups in the primary end point (28-day mortality) or the mean score for organ failure. The rate of serious adverse events was much higher in the intensive-therapy group than in the conventional-therapy group (10.9% versus 5.2%, $P = .01$), however.[102] This result was thought to be related to the very high rate of severe hypoglycemia (serum glucose level, ≥ 40 mg/dL) in the intensive-therapy group (17.0%) as compared with the conventional therapy group (4.1%).[102] The endocrine response to insulin may differ between patients, and normoglycemia can be difficult to achieve safely with insulin; mild hyperglycemia is managed more easily but still requires great vigilance to avoid hypoglycemia.[104]

Emergency Department–Initiated Insulin Protocol in Neurologic Emergencies

Insulin infusion therapy now is used routinely in many medical centers to treat hyperglycemia in critically ill or injured patients. At present, however, such therapy generally is initiated only after transfer from the emergency department to the ICU or, less commonly, to the medical ward. This practice is potentially of concern because it seems to be administratively oriented rather than patient oriented. If rapid and tight glycemic control is beneficial, why should it not be initiated while patients await admission? Insulin protocols may be delayed by hours before patients are transferred from the emergency department to the inpatient unit, and during that time hyperglycemia often is not treated. Then, depending on the protocol used, glycemic control may not be achieved for 8 to 12 hours[84] after initiation of insulin treatment. Efforts to establish a rapidly effective but safe insulin infusion protocol in acutely ill patients in the emergency department have shown promise. A small observational study of patients who were critically ill (as defined by vital signs, an APACHE II score of 9 or higher, the presence of systemic inflammatory response syndrome criteria, or evidence of organ dysfunction) and who had blood glucose levels of 130 mg/dL or higher was performed

Table 3
Blood glucose target levels or range according to source

Location	Blood Glucose Target Level or Range (mg/dL)	
	American Diabetes Association	American College of Endocrinology
ICU	110–180	<110
Medical-surgical unit	90–130, <180 postprandial	<110 before a meal; < 180 maximum

Data from Clement S, Braithwaite SS, Magee MF, et al. Management of diabetes and hyperglycemia in hospitals. Diabetes Care 2004;24:553–91.

to determine the feasibility and safety of intensive insulin therapy to target blood glucose levels between 80 and 110 mg/dL in the emergency department before transfer to a hospital ward or ICU. Target blood glucose levels were achieved within 2.5 to 3 hours after the start of insulin infusion. Only 1 of the 25 patients studied had mild hypoglycemia (blood glucose level < 60 mg/dL) lasting 30 minutes, and none had severe hypoglycemia (blood glucose level < 40 mg/dL or < 60 mg/dL with a change in mental status) (NT Gentile, unpublished results, 2008). This experience suggests that early strict glycemic control is feasible and safe. Intensive bedside resources are needed to reduce and maintain glucose levels between 80 and 110 mg/dL, however. The rate of hypoglycemia can be as high as 16% to 46%,[104] depending on the protocol used. The detrimental effects of hypoglycemia in critical care have been the subject of several recent reports[102–104] and should be avoided conscientiously.

SUMMARY

Early and persistent hyperglycemia can be detrimental in critical illness and injury. Although the role of intensive insulin therapy in acute neuroemergencies has not been established fully, glycemic control is an important adjunct to primary treatment of these disorders. Initiating therapy early after injury is likely to provide the greatest effect on clinical outcome. Perhaps even more than with other acute illness, however, hypoglycemia must be avoided meticulously. Therefore, continued efforts to develop and study the use of safe and reliable protocols to treat hyperglycemia in acute neurologic illness and injury are warranted.

REFERENCES

1. Marr AL, Coronado VG. Central nervous system injury surveillance: annual data submission standards for the year 2002. Atlanta (GA): US Department of Health and Human Services, Centers for Disease Control; 2001.
2. Langlois JA, Rutland-Brown W, Thomas KE. Traumatic brain injury in the United States: emergency department visits, hospitalizations, and deaths. Atlanta (GA): US Department of Health and Human Services, Centers for Disease Control; 2004.
3. CDC. What is traumatic brain injury? Available at: http://www.cdc.gov/node.do/id/0900f3ec8000dbdc. Accessed August 2008.
4. Langlois JA, Kegler SR, Butler JA. Traumatic brain injury-related hospital discharges: results from a 14-state surveillance system, 1997. Atlanta (GA): US Department of Health and Human Services, Centers for Disease Control; 2003. p. 1–18.
5. Coronado VG, Thomas KE. Incidence rates of hospitalization related to traumatic brain injury—12 states, 2002. MMWR 2006;55(08):201–4.
6. Annegers JF, Hauser WA, Coan SP, et al. Population-based study of seizures after traumatic brain injuries. N Engl J Med 1998;338:20–4.
7. Salazar AM, Jabbari B, Vance SC, et al. Epilepsy after penetrating head injury. I. Clinical correlates: a report of the Vietnam head injury study. Neurology 1985;35:1406–14.
8. Cowan LD. The epidemiology of the epilepsies in children. Ment Retard Dev Disabil Res Rev 2002;8(3):171–81.
9. Thomas T, Haase N, Rosamond W, et al. Heart disease and stroke statistics—2006 update. A Report from the American Heart Association Statistics Committee and Stroke Statistics Subcommittee. Circulation 2006;113:e85–151.

10. Murray CJL, Lopez AD. The global burden of disease: a comprehensive assessment of mortality and disability from diseases, injuries, and risk factors in 1990 and projected to 2020. Boston: Harvard University Press; 1996.
11. American Heart Association. Heart disease and stroke statistics—2005 update. Dallas (TX): American Heart Association; 2002.
12. Johnstone B, Price T, Bounds T, et al. Rural/urban differences in vocational outcomes for state vocational rehabilitation clients with TBI. NeuroRehabilitation 2003;18:197–203.
13. CDC. Centers for Disease Control. Available at: http://www.cdc.gov/ncipc/didop/tbi.htm#rate. Accessed August 2008.
14. Sherer M, Nick TG, Sander AM, et al. Race and productivity outcome after traumatic brain injury: influence of confounding factors. J Head Trauma Rehabil. 2003;18(5):408–24.
15. Hart T, Millis S, Novack T, et al. The relationship between neuropsychologic function and level of caregiver supervision at 1 year after traumatic brain injury. Arch Phys Med Rehabil 2003;84(2):221–30.
16. Keppel KG, Pearcy JN, Wagener DK. Trends in racial and ethnic-specific rates for the health status indications: United States, 1990–98. Healthy People 2000 Stat.
17. Weir CJ, Murray GD, Dyker AG, et al. Is hyperglycaemia an independent predictor of poor outcome after acute stroke? Results of a long-term follow-up study. BMJ 1997;314:1303–6.
18. Sacco RL, Boden-Albala B, Abel G, et al. Race-ethnic disparities in the impact of stroke risk factors: the Northern Manhattan Stroke Study. Stroke 2001;32: 1725–31.
19. Brown RD, Whisnant JP, Sicks JD, et al. Stroke incidence, prevalence and survival: secular trends in Rochester, Minnesota through 1989. Stroke 1996;27: 373–80.
20. Broderick J, Brott T, Kothari R, et al. The greater Cincinnati/Northern Kentucky stroke study: preliminary first-ever total incidence rates of stroke among blacks. Stroke 1998;29:415–21.
21. Johnston SC, Fung LH, Gillum LA, et al. Utilization of intravenous tissue-type plasminogen activator for ischemic stroke at academic medical centers: the influence of ethnicity. Stroke 2001;32:1061–8.
22. Gentile NT, Seftchick MW. Poor outcomes in Hispanic and African-American patients after acute ischemic stroke: influence of diabetes and hyperglycemia. Ethn Dis 2008;18:330–5.
23. Cowie CC, Rust KF, Byrd-Holt DD, et al. Prevalence of diabetes and impaired fasting glucose in adults in the US population. National Health and Nutrition Examination Survey 1999–2002. Diabetes Care 2006;29:1263–8.
24. Haire-Joshu D, Fleming C. An ecological approach to understanding contribution to disparities in diabetes prevention and care. Curr Diabetes Rep 2006;6: 123–9.
25. Harris MI, Klein R, Cowie CC, et al. Is the risk of diabetic retinopathy greater in non-Hispanic blacks and Mexican Americans than in non-Hispanic whites with type 2 diabetes: a US population study. Diabetes Care 1998;21:1230–5.
26. Lavery LA, Ashry HR, van Houtum W, et al. Variation in the incidence and proportion of diabetes-related amputations in minorities. Diabetes Care 1996;19: 48–52.
27. Cowie CC, Port FK, Wolfe RA, et al. Disparities in incidence of diabetic end-stage renal disease according to race and type of diabetes. N Engl J Med 1989;321(16):1074–9.

28. Muller B. Endocrine aspects of critical illness. Annee Endocrinol 2007;68: 290–8.
29. Nylen ES, Alarifi AA. Humoral markers of severity and prognosis of critical illness. J Clin Endocrinol Metab 2001;15:553–73.
30. Muller B, Nylen ES. Endocrine changes in critical illness. J Intensive Care Med 2004;19(2):67–82.
31. Capes SE, Hunt D, Malmberg K, et al. Stress hyperglycemia and prognosis of stroke in nondiabetic and diabetic patients: a systematic overview. Stroke 2001;32:2426–32.
32. Williams LS, Rotich J, Qi R, et al. Effects of admission hyperglycemia on mortality and costs in acute ischemic stroke. Neurology 2002;59:67–71.
33. Bruno A, Levine SR, Frankel MR, et al. Admission glucose level and clinical outcomes in the NINDS rt-PA Stroke Trial. Neurology 2002;10(59):669–74.
34. Pulsinelli WA, Levy DE, Sigsbee B, et al. Increased damage after ischemic stroke in patients with hyperglycemia with or without established diabetes mellitus. Am J Med 1983;74:540–4.
35. Berger I, Hakim AM. The association of hyperglycemia with cerebral edema in stroke. Stroke 1986;17:865–71.
36. Bruno A, Biller J, Adams HP Jr, et al. Acute blood glucose level and outcome from ischemic stroke. Neurology 1999;52:280–4.
37. Baird TA, Parsons MW, Phanh T, et al. Persistent poststroke hyperglycemia is independently associated with infarct expansion and worse clinical outcome. Stroke 2003;34:2208–14.
38. de Courten-Myers GM, Kleinholz M, Holm P, et al. Hemorrhagic infarct conversion in experimental stroke. Ann Emerg Med 1992;21:120–6.
39. de Courten-Myers GM, Kleinholz M, Wagner KR, et al. Fatal strokes in hyperglycemic cats. Stroke 1989;20:1707–15.
40. Kawai N, Keep RF, Betz AL. Hyperglycemia and the vascular effects of cerebral ischemia. Stroke 1997;28:149–54.
41. Demchuk AM, Morgenstern LB, Krieger DW, et al. Serum glucose level and diabetes predict tissue plasminogen activator-related intracerebral hemorrhage in acute ischemic stroke. Stroke 1999;30:34–9.
42. Broderick JP, Hagen T, Brott T, et al. Hyperglycemia and hemorrhagic transformation of cerebral infarcts. Stroke 1995;26:484–7.
43. Mitchell AJ. Clinical implications of poststroke hypothalamo-pituitary adrenal axis dysfunction: a critical literature review. J Stroke Cerebrovasc Dis 1997;6: 377–88.
44. O'Neill P, Davies I, Fullerton K, et al. Stress hormone and blood glucose response following acute stroke in the elderly. Stroke 1991;22:842–7.
45. Feibel JH, Hardy PM, Campbell RG, et al. Prognostic value of the stress response following stroke. JAMA 1977;238:1374–7.
46. Prado R, Ginsberg MD, Dietrich WD, et al. Hyperglycemia increases infarct size in collaterally perfused but not end-arterial vascular territories. J Cereb Blood Flow Metab 1988;8:186–92.
47. Acciaressi M, Caso V, Venti M, et al. First-ever stroke and outcome in patients admitted to Perugia stroke unit: predictors for death, dependency, and recurrence of stroke within the first three months. Clin Exp Hypertens 2006; 28(3–4):287–94.
48. Sacco RL, Shi T, Zamanillo MC, et al. Predictors of mortality and recurrence after hospitalized cerebral infarction in an urban community: the Northern Manhattan Stroke Study. Neurology 1994;44:626–34.

49. Soda T, Nakayasu H, Maeda M, et al. Stroke recurrence within the first year following cerebral infarction–Tottori University Lacunar Infarction Prognosis Study (TULIPS). Acat Neurol Scand 2004;110(6):343–9.

50. Megherbi S-E, Milan C, Minier D, et al. Association between diabetes and stroke subtype on survival and functional outcome 3 months after stroke. Data from the European BIOMED Stroke Project. Stroke 2003;34:688–94.

51. Gentile NT, Seftcheck M, Matonti M, et al. Decreased mortality with normalizing blood glucose after acute stroke. Acad Emerg Med 2006;13:174–80.

52. McGirt MJ, Woodworth GF, Ali M, et al. Persistent perioperative hyperglycemia as an independent predictor of poor outcome after aneurysmal subarachnoid hemorrhage. J Neurosurg 2007;107(6):1080–5.

53. Kerner A, Schlenk F, Sakowitz O, et al. Impact of hyperglycemia on neurological deficits and extracellular glucose levels in aneurysmal subarachnoid hemorrhage patients. Neurol Res 2007;29(7):647–53.

54. Srinivasan V, Spinella PC, Drott HR, et al. Association of timing, duration, and intensity of hyperglycemia with intensive care unit mortality in critically ill children. Pediatr Crit Care Med 2004;5:329–36.

55. Branco RG, Garcia PC, Piva JP, et al. Glucose level and risk of mortality in pediatric septic shock. Pediatr Crit Care Med 2005;6:470–2.

56. Powers WJ. Hyperglycemia is not associated with mortality in bacterial meningitis. Ann Neurol 1983;14:82–3.

57. Park WS, Chang YS, Lee M. Effect of induced hyperglycemia on brain cell membrane function and energy metabolism during the early phase of experimental meningitis in newborn piglets. Brain Res 1998;798:195–203.

58. Hoxworth JM, Xu K, Zhou Y, et al. Cerebral metabolic profile, selective neuron loss, and survival of acute and chronic hyperglycemic rats following cardiac arrest and resuscitation. Brain Res 1999;821:467–79.

59. Siesjo BK, Katsura KI, Kristian T, et al. Molecular mechanism of acidosis-mediated damage. Acta Neurochir Suppl (Wien) 1996;66:8–14.

60. Anderson RE, Tan WK, Martin HS, et al. Effects of glucose and PaO2 modulation on cortical intracellular acidosis, NADH redox state, and infarction in the ischemic penumbra. Stroke 1999;30:160–70.

61. Siesjo BK, Zhao Q, Pahlmark K, et al. Glutamate, calcium and free radicals as mediators of ischemic brain damage. Ann Thorac Surg 1995;59:1316–20.

62. Pulsinelli WA, Waldman S, Rawlinson D, et al. Moderate hyperglycemia augments ischemic brain damage: a neuropathologic study in rats. Neurology 1982;32:1239–46.

63. Dietrich WD, Alonso O, Busto R. Moderate hyperglycemia worsens acute blood-brain barrier injury after forebrain ischemia in rats. Stroke 1993;24:111–6.

64. Gentile NT, Vaidyula V, Kanamalla U, et al. Factor VIIa and tissue factor procoagulant activity in diabetes mellitus after acute ischemic stroke: impact of hyperglycemia. Thromb Haemost 2007;98:1007–13.

65. Chaudhuri A, Janicke D, Wilson MF, et al. Anti-inflammatory and profibrinolytic effect of insulin in acute ST-segment-elevation myocardial infarction. Circulation 2004;109(7):849–54.

66. Auer RN. Insulin, blood glucose levels, and ischemic brain damage. Neurology 1998;51(Suppl 3):S39–43.

67. Hui L, Pei DS, Zhang QG, et al. The neuroprotection of insulin on ischemic brain injury in rat hippocampus through negative regulation of JNK signaling pathway by PI3K/Akt activation. Brain Res 2005;1052(1):1–9.

68. Voll CL, Auer RN. Insulin attenuates ischemic brain damage independent of its hypoglycemic effect. J Cereb Blood Flow Metab 1991;11(6):1006–14.
69. Finney SJ, Zekveld C, Elia A, et al. Glucose control and mortality in critically ill patients. JAMA 2003;2190:2041–7.
70. Hamilton MG, Tranmer BI, Auer RN. Insulin reduction of cerebral infarction due to transient focal ischemia. J Neurosurg 1995;82:262–8.
71. LeMay DR, Gehua L, Zelenock GB, et al. Insulin administration protects neurologic function in cerebral ischemia in rats. Stroke 1988;19:1411–9.
72. Van den Berghe G, Wouters P, Weekers F, et al. Intensive insulin therapy in the critically ill patients. N Engl J Med 2001;345(19):1359–67.
73. Van den Berghe G, Wilmer A, Herman H, et al. Intensive insulin therapy in the medical ICU. N Engl J Med 2006;354:449–61.
74. DeSantis AJ, Schmidt K, O'Shea-Mahler E, et al. Inpatient management of hyperglycemia: the Northwestern experience. Endocr Pract 2006;12(5):491–505.
75. Malmberg K. Role of insulin-glucose infusion in outcomes after acute myocardial infarction: the diabetes and insulin-glucose infusion in acute myocardial infarction (DIGAMI) study. Endocr Pract 2004;10(Suppl 2):13–6.
76. Cheung NW, Wong VW, McLean M. The Hyperglycemia: Intensive Insulin Infusion in Infarction (HI-5) Study: a randomized controlled trial of insulin infusion therapy for myocardial infarction. Diabetes Care 2006;29:765–70.
77. Zerr KJ, Furnary AP, Grunkemeier GL, et al. Glucose control lowers the risk of wound infection in diabetics after open heart operations. Ann Thorac Surg 1997;63:356–61.
78. Doenst T, Wijeysundera D, Karkouti K, et al. Hyperglycemia during cardiopulmonary bypass is an independent risk factor for mortality in patients undergoing cardiac surgery. J Thorac Cardiovasc Surg 2005;130:1144.
79. Furnary AP, Zerr KJ, Grunkemeier GL, et al. Hyperglycemia: a predictor of mortality following CABG in diabetics. Circulation 1999;100(Suppl):1–591.
80. Furnary AP, Gao G, Grunkemeier GL, et al. Continuous insulin infusion reduces mortality in patients with diabetes undergoing coronary artery bypass grafting. J Thorac Cardiovasc Surg 2003;125:1007–21.
81. Malmberg K, Rydén L, Hamsten A, et al. Effects of insulin treatment on cause-specific one-year mortality and morbidity in diabetic patients with acute myocardial infarction. Eur Heart J 1996;17:1337–44.
82. Malmberg K, DIGAMI study group. Prospective randomised study of intensive insulin treatment on long term survival after acute myocardial infarction in patients with diabetes mellitus. BMJ 1997;314:1512–5.
83. Malmberg K. Intense metabolic control by means of insulin in patients with diabetes mellitus and acute myocardial infarction (DIGAMI 2): effects on mortality and morbidity. Eur Heart J 2005;26:650–61.
84. Pinto A, Skolnick A, Kirtane S, et al. U-shaped relationship of blood glucose with adverse outcomes among patients with ST-segment elevation myocardial infarction. J Am Coll Cardiol 2005;46:178–80.
85. Sung J, Bochicchio GV, Joshi MM, et al. Admission hyperglycemia is predictive of outcome in critically ill trauma patients. J Trauma 2005;59:1353–8.
86. Scalea TM, Bochicchio GV, Bochicchio KM, et al. Tight glycemic control in critically injured trauma patients. Ann Surg 2007;246(4):605–10 [discussion: 610–2].
87. Van den Berghe G, Schoonheydt K, Becx P, et al. Insulin therapy protects the central and peripheral nervous system of intensive care patients. Neurol 2005; 64:1348–53.

88. Jeremitsky E, Omert L, Dunham CM, et al. Harbingers of poor outcome the day after severe brain injury: hypothermia, hypoxia, and hypoperfusion. J Trauma 2003;54:312–9.

89. Young B, Ott L, Dempsey R, et al. Relationship between admission hyperglycemia and neurologic outcome of severely brain-injured patients. Ann Surg 1989;210:466–72.

90. Vespa P, Boonyaputthikul R, McArthur DL, et al. Intensive insulin therapy reduces microdialysis glucose values without altering glucose utilization or improving the lactate/pyruvate ratio after traumatic brain injury. Crit Care Med 2006;34(3):850–6.

91. Voll C, Auer R. The effect of postischemic blood glucose levels on ischemic brain damage in the rat. Ann Neurol 1988;24:638–46.

92. Ginsberg MD, Prado R, Dietrich WD, et al. Hyperglycemia reduces the extent of cerebral infarction in rats. Stroke 1987;18:570–4.

93. Kraft SA, Larson CP Jr, Shuer LM, et al. Effect of hyperglycemia on neuronal changes in a rabbit model of focal cerebral ischemia. Stroke 1990;21:447–50.

94. Scott JF, Robinson GM, French JM, et al. Glucose potassium insulin infusions in the treatment of acute stroke patients with mild to moderate hyperglycemia. Stroke 1999;30:793–9.

95. Gray CS, Hildreth AJ, Sandercock PA, et al. Glucose-potassium-insulin infusions in the management of post-stroke hyperglycemia: the UK glucose insulin in stroke trial (GIST-UK). Lancet Neurol 2007;6:397–406.

96. McCormick Mt, Muir KW, Gray CS, et al. Management of hyperglycemia in stroke. Stroke 2008;39:2177–85.

97. Walters MR, Weir CJ, Lees K. A randomised, controlled pilot study to investigate the potential benefit of intervention with insulin in hyperglycemic acute ischemic stroke patients. Cerebrovasc Dis 2006;22:116–22.

98. Bruno A, Saha C, Williams LS, et al. IV insulin during acute cerebral infarction in diabetic patients. Neurol 2004;62:1441–2.

99. Johnston KC. Glucose regulation in acute stroke patients trial. Available at: https://grasptrial.org/grasp/home.aspx. Accessed May 2, 2008.

100. Bruno A, Kent TA, Coull BM, et al. Treatment of hyperglycemia in ischemic stroke (THIS). Stroke 2008;39:384–9.

101. Wilson M, Weinreb J, Hoo GWS. Intensive insulin therapy in critical care: a review of 12 protocols. Diabetes Care 2007;30:1005–11.

102. Brunkhorst FM, Engel C, Bloos F, et al. Intensive insulin therapy and pentastarch resuscitation in severe sepsis. N Engl J Med 2008;358:125–39.

103. Clement S, Braithwaite SS, Magee MF, et al. Management of diabetes and hyperglycemia in hospitals. Diabetes Care 2004;24:553–91.

104. Freire AX, Avecillas JF, Yataco JC, et al. Hypoglycemia risk: a cause for concern in the intensive care unit hyperglycemia control debate. Crit Care Med 2007;35(4):1222.

Index

Note: Page numbers of article titles are in **boldface** type.

Emerg Med Clin N Am 27 (2009) 171–178
doi:10.1016/S0733-8627(09)00010-8
0733-8627/09/$ – see front matter © 2009 Elsevier Inc. All rights reserved.

emed.theclinics.com

Moving?

Make sure your subscription moves with you!

To notify us of your new address, find your **Clinics Account Number** (located on your mailing label above your name), and contact customer service at:

E-mail: elspcs@elsevier.com

800-654-2452 (subscribers in the U.S. & Canada)
314-453-7041 (subscribers outside of the U.S. & Canada)

Fax number: 314-523-5170

Elsevier Periodicals Customer Service
11830 Westline Industrial Drive
St. Louis, MO 63146

*To ensure uninterrupted delivery of your subscription, please notify us at least 4 weeks in advance of move.

ELSEVIER

Printed and bound by CPI Group (UK) Ltd, Croydon, CR0 4YY

03/10/2024

01040445-0016